Pregnancy Diary

A Christian Mother's Reflections

Mary Arnold

Pregnancy Diary

A Christian Mother's Reflections

IGNATIUS PRESS   SAN FRANCISCO

Cover design by Riz Boncan Marsella
Cover art by Chris Pelicano

© 1996 Ignatius Press, San Francisco
All rights reserved
ISBN 0–89870–564–9
Library of Congress catalogue number 95–79887
Printed in the United States of America ∞

To God the Father, the Creator of all life—

"You it was who created my inmost self,
and put me together in my mother's womb;
for all these mysteries I thank you:
for the wonder of myself,
   for the wonder of your works."

Psalm 138

Contents

Foreword 9

The First Trimester 13

The Second Trimester 53

The Third Trimester 95

Conclusion 145

Postscript 149

Foreword

Before I begin, a word of thanks to my dear and long-suffering husband, Edmund, for putting up with what he terms "The Craziness" I exhibit when pregnant and nursing a newborn. I apologize for being crazy, but if I stitched a watermelon into his abdomen and injected a riot of hormones into his veins, he might go crazy, too. Pregnancy, for all its joys, is hard work. I once read a book by a doctor who worked at Childrens' Hospital in San Francisco. The doctor claimed that a woman's body is superior to a man's because it is biologically more complex (in that she has menstrual cycles, she carries the baby, she nurses). Any man knows that the more complex and finely tuned the vehicle, the more temperamental it is. If the man is a Chevy truck, the woman is a Lambourghini. If pregnant women rant and rave, it is because we are masterpieces of creation.

A word of thanks, too, to my wonderful parents in New Zealand, who endowed their seven children with a great respect for human life and with a love of babies. My dad was an obstetrician who delivered over fifteen thousand babies before retiring at age seventy. He started the prolife movement in New Zealand. He is one of the most gracious, loving and courageous men I know and has a delightful sense of humor as well. And thanks to my mother, the heart of the family. And what a beautiful, generous heart she has.

So why another pregnancy book?

I didn't plan this book. It began to fall out of me the day after I discovered I was pregnant. "Pregnancy", according to the dictionary, is a time of being filled up with new life. But it also means: "teeming with ideas, imaginative, inventive, fruitful".

That's how I have always felt when pregnant. Other moms experience the same thing. Not only are our wombs full and pulsating with new life, but our heads are full of thoughts of the future: What if? What when? What will this child be? What will his future hold? Insomnia in early pregnancy is usually blamed on hormones. In my own experience I find it mainly occurs because one's head teems with ideas, excitement, questions—none of which helps one to fall asleep quickly.

I believe that, to millions of women, pregnancy and childbirth are deeply spiritual experiences. When we become pregnant, our thoughts turn inward and upward. We are filled with awe at what is happening in the limbo of our wombs, where the baby is being silently knitted together. This wonderful act of creation is within us but independent of us. We appreciate more than any other time that God exists; that he loves us and blesses us with new life; that he is in control of the pregnancy. I believe this experience is common to all pregnant women who have religious faith. Pregnancy brings us closer to God. Just as our physical juices flow strongly in pregnancy, so do our spiritual juices.

Yet there are no books that testify to this religious experience. In my first week of being pregnant, I went to my local library to see what was available on the subject of pregnancy. Most books were on the subjects of health, nutrition, exercises (Jane Fonda's pregnancy workout book—thanks, but no thanks), problems during pregnancy, Lamaze and breathing, the delivery, etc. But nothing personal. Then I did find a book that looked personal: *What Only a Mother Can Tell You about Having a Baby*, written by a former assistant editor for *Newsday* and published in 1980. "This sounds good", I thought. But the book started out in a vulgar, smart-alecky tone with sexual jokes and negative, feminist comments about pregnancy. Women interviewed talked about "not using rubbers" and why morning sickness had led them to have abortions. The book didn't appeal to me.

I am Catholic, and my book will be written from a Christian woman's perspective, which views pregnancy as a blessing, not a curse; a gift to be accepted in spite of the hardships it brings, not a disease to be terminated by abortion. This positive view of pregnancy will accord with the views of all women, Christian or non-Christian, who accept God as the Creator and life as sacred.

Because (God willing) I will deliver this baby at age forty-two, my observations may be useful to that growing number of American women carrying babies in their late thirties and early forties—the so-called "dangerous time". Pregnant women over thirty-five are subject to a barrage of "genetic counseling" and almost forced to undergo amniocentesis. Christian women need to know that if they oppose abortion, all this counseling is a waste of time, and amniocentesisis is dangerous for the baby. But more about that later.

Women love to talk. Pregnant women especially love to talk with other pregnant women, sharing their common experiences, joys, pains, fears and hopes as the baby grows. This little weekly diary will be a companion. It is a book in which you can trace the progress of my pregnancy, and it will be interesting to compare whether you are experiencing the same aches and pains, cramps, fears, delights, movements, etc., and at what stage these things occur. I believe that some stay-at-home moms are lonely in today's neighborhoods, where all the other mothers have left for work by 7:30 A.M. Some pregnant moms are starved for company. For them, this book might provide companionship.

The First Trimester

We begin our diary at week five of pregnancy because week four or five is when the mother discovers she is pregnant. To make it easy, however, obstetricians calculate a pregnancy from the beginning of the last menstrual period, i.e., before the woman is even pregnant. Using this date, pregnancy lasts about 280 days, or forty weeks.

WEEK FIVE

Saturday, October 2, 1993

Being overdue by one day, I took my temperature this morning, and it was 98.6. Could this mean I'm pregnant? Usually if I go a day late, my temp will already be dropping and in the 97-to-97.5 range. By 4 P.M. today, I feel sleepy and wonder if this, too, might be a sign.

Sunday, October 3

Today when I awake I take my temp again. It is 98.6 degrees. This must be it. After more than four years of waiting and praying for another baby, it looks as if I might be pregnant.

What makes me especially hopeful is a strange experience. When my husband was laid off from his job as a construction project manager a month ago, a friend sent us a beautiful card about Saint Thérèse of Lisieux (otherwise known as the Little Flower). At the time I knew little about this saint, who was a Carmelite nun and died at the tender age of twenty-four. Nevertheless, reading the card, I found that Thérèse had promised to "spend my heaven doing good on earth" and that on her deathbed she promised "to let fall a shower of roses on the earth". Many Catholics pray to Saint Thérèse, and they say she sends them a rose and helps them. I didn't pay much attention to the card, because I had practically given up hope of ever conceiving another child (my three children are Luke, 9; Laura, 7; Hannah, 6). But I did ask Saint Thérèse to ask Jesus if he would send me another baby. "And if he says Yes, send me a rose", I prayed. I told no one of this prayer, but a week later Hannah gave me a white piece of paper onto which she had taped bright red rose petals to form the shape of a flower. It was lovely, and I pinned it on my bedroom wall. "Is this the rose?" I wondered but didn't hold out much hope.

Then on October 1, my period was due (I am on a regular twenty-six-day cycle). The priest at that morning's Mass announced that it was the feast of Saint Thérèse, the Little Flower. I was surprised to hear this! I thought it might be significant. Now, on my second day of having a high temperature, I wonder if Saint Thérèse is answering my prayers. . . .

I feel so strangely confident that I have conceived, I get out of bed and prostrate myself on the floor, praying, "Thank you, Father; thank you, Son; thank you, Holy Spirit."

I go to the supermarket and buy an "Answer" pregnancy kit. (At eight dollars, it is the cheapest I can find.) Back home, while my husband cooks bacon and eggs, the test paper in the kit turns pink.

"I'm pregnant!" I tell Ed. He takes me in his arms in a bear hug. I appreciate his hug and his generosity. So many of my friends' husbands don't want more than two children, and I can relate to how they feel, because it is hard to exist these days on a single income. I am glad that Ed can see the value of another baby in spite of the fact we are always short of cash. As the children come downstairs, sleepily rubbing their eyes, we give them the good news. Mom is pregnant! They are thrilled and start talking into my tummy button, welcoming the baby.

We head off to Sunday Mass. At Communion time all I can say is "Thank you. Thank you. Thank you." I am embarrassed to find tears running down my cheeks.

Monday, October 4

We call my dad in New Zealand to tell him the good news. He and Mom are thrilled, but he cautions me that it's too early to trust the home test and to wait longer. "The home tests are only 70 percent accurate", he warns.

Dad is an old-fashioned obstetrician, who prefers to

tell the woman she is pregnant rather than the other way around. Nevertheless, he is an excellent doctor, so his remark unnerves me to the point that I go to the market and purchase a second, more expensive ($14.95) test, "E.P.T.", by a different manufacturer. This one is simpler. You hold a stick under your urine stream for five seconds, and in four minutes you have your answer—pregnant or not pregnant. It's positive. I like proving obstetricians wrong!

Tuesday, October 5

Temp still nice and high—98.3 this morning.

How does one feel in early pregnancy? Prior to missing my period, I had felt premenstrual in the sense that my womb was "full", as it feels before you bleed. I even felt a single cramp two days before due date. I still have that feeling of puffiness, being filled up, heavy and . . . pregnant. I have achiness around the abdominal area but no further cramping sensation, as when the womb contracts to force out the menstrual flow. Some women complain of cramps after they are pregnant, and this always poses concern about whether they will miscarry.

Wednesday, October 6

Temp this morn is 98.5, so I'm still pregnant. The temperature is very reliable, as those who use the Sympto-Thermal method of Natural Family Planning know. Although the temperature shift is only slight, it is an accurate indicator. The temperature drops steadily as menstruation approaches. Most obstetricians will tell you if your temperature is high on your menstrual due date, you are probably pregnant. I know for a fact I would never bleed on a day when my temperature is this high.

Thursday, October 7

Temp 98.6.

How am I feeling physically? Most women complain of tiredness in the first trimester of pregnancy. I still feel tired by early afternoon and sometimes lie down around 2 P.M., just before I have to pick up the kids from school. This rest energizes me for the busy afternoon of helping with homework, getting dinner, dishes, bathtime and the almighty assault involved in getting three children to go to bed.

How about psychologically? I always suffer from stress during pregnancy, and I am definitely snapping at the children, less patient than usual. Little things make me react sharply—unfortunately for the kids and Ed. Ed thinks I go mad during pregnancy. Well, that's not altogether true. He regards me as slightly maniacal at the best of times! During pregnancy, he says, my mania becomes more profound. This evening he frowned at me when I pointed to my stomach and said, "Kiss your baby good night."

"Oh, no", he groaned. "The craziness begins!"

Friday, October 8

Three days ago I started taking prenatal vitamins—"Professional Prenatal Formula by Lifetime", which I got at the local health-food store. These are the prenatal tablets recommended by Marilyn Shannon in her book *Fertility, Cycles, and Nutrition* (1990, published by The Couple to Couple League, P.O. Box 111184, Cincinnati, Ohio 45211).

Shannon writes, "These are the best prenatal pills available as this book goes to press" (p. 95). How do these differ from the ones your doctor would prescribe? They are much higher in vitamin B_6—which Shannon considers essential in combatting edema (swelling) in pregnancy. Also higher in magnesium and calcium. You take six a day, which is a bore, but Shannon and others say this is more effective, nutritionally, than popping just the one heavy-duty pill in the morning.

Most obstetricians won't mind if you ask to use these vitamins instead of the prescription ones. But do check that your doctor considers these vitamins safe, because an overdose of certain vitamins can be harmful to the fetus. These "lifetime" vitamins cost fifteen dollars a month, which adds up to about $135 for the nine months—and more if you continue to take them while nursing. But it is an investment in your and your baby's good health, and pregnancy is definitely a nutritional stress on the body.

I was impressed with Shannon's book because of

the statistics she gives showing how vitamins can help with infertility, premenstrual syndrome and also with numerous problems in pregnancy—mask of pregnancy, edema, eclampsia, etc. Also, it is now widely recognized that folic acid, taken in the preconceptual and early days of pregnancy, is effective in helping prevent spina bifida and related defects. Because Shannon provided statistics, I finally stopped being cynical about vitamins and started taking 200 mg of B_6 daily about three weeks before I found I was pregnant. (B_6 seems to be something of a wonder drug for infertility and pregnancy problems.) The B_6 may have helped me, but I still believe it is always God who either wills the baby or does not will it. At my age I have to work harder at being healthy, so I'll take all the supplements I can get. So far, I feel great.

Week Six

How is the baby doing?

The baby's heart is already beating and has been doing so since twenty-one days after conception. It is a rudimentary heart in the sense that it has only two chambers, as opposed to the four that a fully grown heart has. Nevertheless, it is interesting to think that about the time a mother discovers she is pregnant, her baby's heart is already beating! I have a bumper sticker on my car that reads "Abortion stops a beating heart"—and it always does. The baby now has the rudiments of eyes, ears and a mouth. Little buds of tissue have formed where the arms and legs will subsequently develop.

To get to this stage, the embryonic baby had to make a perilous journey down the fallopian tube (where fertilization took place) and into the womb, where he attached himself to the spongy lining of the uterine wall. From a few hundred cells in the first week of life, he increased to many thousands of cells in this first month. This represents the most prodigious growth rate in the child's life!

Saturday, October 9

I recently started using the breviary, the Church's daily prayer book, which is full of Psalms and Scripture readings, organized on a daily basis. Wednesday's Canticle of Judith (excerpts from Chapter 16) was particularly poignant in my pregnant state:

> Strike up the instruments,
> a song to my God with timbrels,
> chant to the Lord with cymbals.
> Sing to him a new song,
> exalt and acclaim his name.
>
> A new hymn I will sing to my God. . . .
> Let your every creature serve you;
> for you spoke, and they were made,

you sent forth your spirit, and they were created;
no one can resist your word.

Thank you, Father, for the new life within me. Please cherish and protect it. Knit it together in secret in the limbo of my womb. I entrust this baby to you.

Sunday, October 10

Infertility is a problem today with women, partly because of sexual liberation, which takes a toll on a woman's body and renders her less capable of conceiving, and partly because of prolonged contraceptive use. The Pill and IUD can wreak havoc with a woman's fertility, and often women are not warned of the dangers to their fertility by enthusiastic obstetricians who prescribe these things too easily. I feel sorry for women who are suffering through infertility. The desire for a baby is so powerful that if it is not met, the sadness can be intense. In Genesis 30:1, Rachel tells Jacob, "Give me children, or I shall die!"

I found that after two or three years of being unable to conceive (although I had previously borne three children, and my doctor told me there was nothing physically wrong with me), I gradually came to accept God's will. Yet I started out impatient and even angry with him.

We go with a local priest, Father Terry Tompkins, once a week to an abortion clinic to pray and offer alternatives to the women going in. One day I watched these poor women, looking so sad and distressed, carrying their babies past me to their deaths. I thought, "Lord, you could have put that baby in my womb. Why did you put him in her womb, knowing that he would end up in Dr. ——'s suction machine?" But, as a girlfriend pointed out to me, "God's ways are not our ways."

Still I looked green-eyed at every pregnant woman in the supermarket. Gradually, I came to accept his will and even to praise him for it, as the Bible instructs us to praise God in all situations. I thought, "If that is what he wants, I'll praise him." This led to the comical situation of my muttering on the day my period began, "Praise you, Lord, for my empty womb. Praise you, Lord, for this wonderful empty womb. Thy will be done." Stupid, isn't it? And yet it helped me to feel happy in God's will and to trust that he knew best.

Monday, October 11

Although I gave up praying for a baby, my children did not. Sometimes while praying the rosary at night (on those nights we managed it, and we do not always get around to it), I would ask the kids what they wanted to pray for. Inevitably, the three of them would chirp: "For a baby." "Oh, quit with the baby stuff", I'd tell them. "There are more important things to pray for. We can't spend all our time on babies. Let's leave that to God." But they ignored me and prayed for a baby anyway.

In fact, one day Laura (seven) told me she was definitely *not* going to stop asking God for a baby. The children are in public school, but I teach them religion at home from the Ignatius Press Faith and Life series. Laura read in one of her lessons about prayer: "Ask, and you shall receive; seek, and you shall find."

"That's what God said to do, and I'm doing it", she said, stubbornly. Laura is a thin, pretty, feminine little girl, but beneath this deceptive exterior lies a steely spirit.

"Well, Lord, you've unleashed a tiger here", I thought. "You had better keep your word now. Anyway ... how can you resist the faith of a little child?"

Tuesday, October 12

Recently I read in the breviary (from Psalm 34):

> Revere the Lord, you his saints.
> They lack nothing, those who revere him.
> Strong lions suffer want and go hungry
> but those who seek the Lord lack no blessing.

And what is a baby, if not a blessing?

Father Richard Roach, a Jesuit moral theologian, once explained to me how God is our "Father" because the nature of the masculine is to create life *outside* of himself, and God created the world separate, independent, outside of himself. The Church, on the other hand, is referred to in feminine terms because the Church nourishes life *within* herself. Inside the womb of the Church are the souls whom she works to educate, sanctify, purify and nurture. Which is better, I wonder?

Certainly the masculine is more dramatic—the male literally pours life out of himself. How wonderful and powerful. But the female nurtures that life within. It is not dramatic, this female procreating. It is invisible, silent, quiet . . . overlooked. The woman builds in darkness. This makes feminists angry. Are they jealous of the male role? But the long, hard work of invisible nurturing is also precious. While the male's role might conjure up adjectives like "power", "speed", "vitality", the woman's role is evocative of "tenderness", "patience", "fortitude".

Wednesday, October 13

So far, no nausea. I don't usually feel very sick in pregnancy, and it usually takes a few weeks before nausea hits. I read that vitamins may help alleviate morning sickness, and so far I feel fine, apart from a little breast tenderness and sleepiness in the afternoons.

"I don't want our baby to look like a hot dog", complains Luke. We have been looking at the beautiful *Life* photos (August 1990 issue), taken by Lennart Nilsson, showing sperm fertilization, the blastocyst passing through the tube into the uterus and then the gradual development of the embryo.

Luke need not worry. The baby has already changed from a plain, elongated shape (like a hot dog) into a more complex shape, where an early eye is discernible, as well as vertebrae. The rudimentary heart is already pumping.

I cannot visit an obstetrician yet, as Ed recently changed jobs, and the new insurance company tells me I cannot be seen until after the insurance kicks in, or the pregnancy will be considered a "pre-existing condition". In the next week or two I shall visit the doctor.

I should mention here that it's a good idea for women to have their minister or priest bless the baby in utero. The Catholic Church has an official Blessing of Women in Pregnancy. One of the prayers from this blessing reads: "Lord God . . . , you made John the Baptist to be filled with the Holy Spirit and leap in his mother's womb, accept the sacrifice of a contrite heart and the fervent prayer of your handmaid, N——, who humbly beseeches you for the preservation of the offspring which you have given her to conceive.

"Take care of this daughter of yours and defend her from the snares and malice of the devil that, by the hand of your mercy, her child may come happily to the light of day and may be preserved for holy baptism, may always serve you in all things and may merit to attain everlasting life."

Thursday, October 14

I was awakened last night from a deep sleep by the need to empty my bladder. The baby presses on the bladder in early pregnancy and then again in the ninth month, so that one feels the need to urinate every hour.

When I move suddenly in bed (when I roll over, for instance), I get a muscular pain in the area of the womb, but I still feel fine and no morning sickness.

The kids are fighting over whether we should have a boy or a girl. Ed and Luke favor a boy, *naturellement*, and the girls want another girl. The names we favor are: boys—Sebastian, Samuel, Stephen, Jacob, Sean, Gabriel, Damien, Tobias, Dominic, John and Thomas; girls—Elizabeth, Rachel, Monica, Maria, Emily, Sarah, Sophie, Victoria, Heather, Veronica, Grace and Kate.

For a boy we have settled on Samuel Thomas. (I am happy with this because, in the Book of Samuel, his mother, Hannah, prayed for a long time to conceive, and when he was born she said, "I will call him Samuel because I asked God for him.") Like Hannah, I spent a long time asking God for this baby.

Friday, October 15

I spoke too soon about not being nauseated. Morning sickness struck this morning—not vomiting, just a general queasiness that left me groaning as I prepared the kids' breakfast.

Sleepiness persists. I am fine in the mornings, but around 2 or 3 P.M. I need to lie down for a half hour. I was never like this before conceiving. I was the one still banging around the house at 11 P.M., putting off going to bed. Now I crawl into bed at 9 P.M. I awoke the past few nights around 3 A.M. to relieve my bladder.

Week Seven

Sunday, October 17

I love the questions children ask. Over the past few years we have lit candles in church to ask our Blessed Mother for a baby.

"Are we going to tell Sam we spent a fortune on candles to get him?" Laura asks this morning as we drive home.

We pass a car with an "Impeach Clinton" bumper sticker. "What does 'impeach' mean?" asks Hannah. "Does it mean they tie him to a tree and throw cans of peaches at him?"

"No," I tell her, "but it's a nice idea."

This week Hannah asked me, "Do you ever think about buying a turtle, Mom?" and "Do princesses wear socks?"

Tuesday, October 19

The last two days my nausea has been worse, although I have not actually vomited. Mothers always comfort one another on this score by saying, "Well, that's a good sign. All your hormones must be working." This may or may not be true, but when you smell bacon cooking and run to the bathroom to gag, it's small comfort.

I brought home from the library a book with the title *Pregnancy after 35*, by Carole Spearin McCauley (New York: Dutton, 1976). I feared it would have a lot of dire tales about the disasters befalling older mothers. In fact, it contained some cheerful news. The author cites a study of twenty-six mothers aged over forty-five who delivered from 1957 to 1971 at Strong Memorial Hospital, Rochester, New York. The analysis was done by Dr. Robert Sokol and associates and reported in the *American Journal of Obstetrics and Gynecology* (1974) 119:6. Some of his conclusions are:

> The woman over 45 tends to be generally healthy. There are no important differences in antepartum and postpartum complications when compared to younger patients of similar parity.
>
> Advanced obstetrical age is not associated with labor prolongation, but the risk of abnormal labor progression (due mostly to malposition) is significantly increased. 50% of the (older) group experienced an abnormal labor (vs. 16% of the young control group) .

> Anesthesia in both groups was minimal. Approximately 85% of patients in both groups (i.e., young and old) received no more than nitrous oxide and a pudendal block. No caudal anesthesia was used. . . . The father of one healthy infant was 75 years old!

Spearin McCauley continues,

> Dr. Albert Hayden, a Teaneck, New Jersey, obstetrician, is an optimist on the question of late pregnancy. "It's more of a pleasure to take care of a woman having her first baby at 40 because it is a very exciting time of her life. She makes a good patient and the reason is that she has had 40 years to mature." After studying 600 mothers over 40, he concluded that while there are a few more problems, "older women do seek prenatal care. They are probably attended more carefully, and they make more visits to the obstetrician than the younger age group."
>
> Dr. Hayden also admits a personal bias. "My mother was 47 years old when I was born, so I am all for women over 40 having babies" (p. 19).

While these were nice anecdotes, a lot of the book deals with genetic counseling and encourages women to abort defective babies. I didn't find any pregnancy book that opposed abortion.

Friday, October 22

The past two days I've felt particularly nauseous in the mornings but not so bad at night—classic morning sickness, I guess, but no vomiting.

Still very sleepy in the afternoons. I cannot believe the drowsiness that accompanies pregnancy. One goes from feeling energetic and able to dance the night away to feeling completely listless. Who would believe a tiny five-week-old baby could have such an effect on the body?

I was telling a thirty-year-old mother of five how tired I felt.

"It must be because I'm forty-one, and the body is not so handy at carrying a baby", I said.

"No, I always sleepwalk through the first trimester of my pregnancies", she replied.

This made me feel better.

Week Eight

Tuesday, October 26

My first visit to the obstetrician. I must say, being from New Zealand, I have a rather jaundiced view of American obstetricians, because here, since so many Americans sue their doctors, the doctors practice "defensive medicine", and the patient often loses out. What do I mean by this?

I mean that when one has a baby in New Zealand or Australia, the doctor has a much lower cesarean rate (10 percent, compared with 20 to 25 percent in

America). Foreign doctors are more prepared to use forceps, to do an external version (turning a breech baby into the correct head-down position) or to deliver a breech birth. All of these things help the mother avoid major surgery. But in America, because of the huge amount of litigation, doctors have adopted a hands-off policy. There is little the doctor will do to help the mother deliver vaginally. If she has problems, the only solution is to slice her open and take the baby. This makes the doctor's job easy but the mother's more difficult. If this happens in a first delivery, then the woman has a weak point on her uterus (the scar) that could rupture in a subsequent labor. Hence the policy in America used to be: "Once a cesarean, always a cesarean." But in the past ten years, insurance companies have protested the high costs of surgical deliveries, so now an increasing number of obstetricians will allow the mom to try for a vaginal delivery after a prior cesarean.

This happened with me. I had a c-section for my first baby and have had two vaginal births since. Obviously, I hope this baby will also be a vaginal birth.

My cynicism about American obstetrics was not eased when the first thing the nurse gave me was a "Patient-Physician Arbitration Agreement", which I was asked to sign and return to the office on my next visit. The gist of the statement was that the patient would promise not to go to court to sue but would allow a medical arbitration group to decide a dispute. I resented being handed this document, and, after consulting with Ed, we decided not to sign it. Not that we have ever sued anyone, but we are not anxious to sign away our legal rights. This sort of unpleasant experience would never happen in most other Western countries.

When the nurse called me into the doctor's office, she took my blood pressure and the date of my last period and then immediately said, "Because of your advanced age, we recommend genetic testing and amniocentesis."

"I'm not having either", I told her. Nevertheless, she gave me three documents about detection of birth defects to take home and read. The birth defects targeted by genetic counselors are Down's syndrome, hemophilia, sickle-cell anemia, cystic fibrosis and neural-tube defects such as spina bifida.

The pamphlets suggest either amniocentesis between weeks fifteen and twenty or chorionic villus sampling between weeks nine and twelve of pregnancy. What the doctor does not tell you is that, if a defect is suspected, nothing can be done to help the baby at this stage. The only "treatment" offered would be abortion. This is why prolife mothers should refuse all of these tests.

The word "abortion" is not mentioned in the pamphlet, which simply states, "If the woman feels it is best, she may choose not to continue the pregnancy." This is a euphemism for a saline abortion, where the baby's skin will be pickled and burned by an injection of salt solution, and, after thrashing in pain for twenty-four hours, the dying baby will initiate labor, and the mother will deliver her dead, defective baby. Of course, sometimes the amniocentesis will give a false positive, and the mom will deliver a perfectly normal but now dead and burned baby. So much for genetic diagnosis and treatment!

From the nurse I proceed to the doctor's room for an interview. I shall not name the doctor, or I would not be able to write honestly. He is affable and does not do abortions, though he does offer contraception and sterilization. The doctor congratulates me on being pregnant, discusses diet and exercise, etc. Then he also mentions amniocentesis. Thanks, but no thanks, I tell him. At this point, he tells me, "Your baby has a one in nineteen chance of being Down's syndrome."

"I thought it was one in forty", I reply.

"At age forty it is that. But you will deliver at age forty-two, so the likelihood increases", says the doctor.

"Well, so be it. That is God's decision, not mine."

Months after this visit with my doctor I came across a book, *The ACOG Guide to Planning for Pregnancy, Birth, and Beyond*, published in 1990 by The American College of Obstetricians and Gynecologists, which states that a forty-two-year-old woman has a one in sixty-three chance of having a Down's syndrome baby (p. 68). This is much better odds than my obstetrician was giving me. For a twenty-year-old, the risk is one in 1,667; for a thirty-year-old, one in 952; at thirty-five, one in 378; at forty, one in 106; at forty-five, one in thirty. Although the figure decreases with age, the fact remains that a woman in her forties has a pretty good chance of having a normal baby. Wouldn't it be refreshing to find an obstetrician who would tell her that!

The truth is that in the game of childbearing there are no guarantees, nor should we ask for any. Who is to say that our physically perfect baby might not turn into a morally deformed teenager or a goddess-worshipping feminist in her twenties? Who is to say that a physically handicapped infant might not be the one who eventually saves other members of the family through her prayers? We can't give the Almighty prerequisites for our children. Life is a dangerous game. We just have to take a deep breath and muddle on through.

What the doctors do not spell out is that amniocentesis also carries a risk of miscarriage. Some mothers carrying very much wanted babies have lost the babies as a direct result of having amniocentesis. In fact, my father, H. P. Dunn, in his book *The Doctor and Christian Marriage* (Staten Island, New York: Alba House, 1992), describes a case where a woman, aged forty, was thrilled to conceive but was talked into amniocentesis by two professors. She underwent the procedure and as a result miscarried a perfectly healthy baby. She was not able to conceive again.

In addition, he points out that, worldwide, the reported incidence of miscarriage after amniocentesis is about 5 percent and after chorionic villus sampling is slightly higher. In other words, the risks of the diagnostic procedure are greater than incidence of fetal abnormality. Moreover, according to the Medical Research Council in London, the simple insertion of the needle and taking out of some fluid carries its own risks: needle-stick injuries to the baby, prematurity, respiratory distress, orthopedic defects, etc.

I ask my doctor whether he will turn a breech baby (external version), as I do not want to have a cesarean if the baby is the wrong way round. He says he will not, because I have already had one cesarean, and an external version could rupture the scar. He says, however, that maybe someone at Stanford University Medical School would turn the baby if it were found to be breech. Here again, this differs from many other countries, where most doctors would not hesitate to turn a breech baby, regardless of whether the mother had had a prior cesarean.

Here I must report an amusing story. When I was eight months pregnant with my second baby, my father was visiting us and discovered the baby was breech. Fearing my doctor would perform a cesarean, he turned the baby himself. This was a simple procedure. I lay on the couch, and Dad placed his fingers on my abdomen and applied pressure, guiding the baby to a head-down position. It took about five minutes. The baby remained head down, and I had an easy, drug-free delivery. But I could never tell my obstetrician that my dad had intervened, because his actions were, strictly speaking, "unethical", considering I was not his patient.

My doctor gives me a physical check-up and tells me to report back in four weeks.

That night in my breviary I read from Revelation (4:11),

> O Lord, our God, you are worthy
> to receive glory and honor and power.
> For you have created all things;
> by your will they came to be and were made.

Yes, Lord, it is by your will that my baby came to be. If he is less than perfect, then that is your will, too, and we will love and cherish him as though he were as perfect as my other children. You yourself supply the strength.

While Down's syndrome persons are very much the object of obstetricians' "search and destroy" techniques, it's worth remembering that they are a peaceful, law-abiding section of our society. One never reads of Down's-syndrome persons bombing the World Trade Center or kidnapping and murdering little children or mowing down diners at McDonald's with a machine gun. I can't recall ever reading anything bad about any Down's-syndrome child, so why are we determined to exterminate this segment of the population?

Week Nine

Tuesday, November 2

Today I visited a chic maternity boutique, Pea in a Pod. I am astounded by the price of maternity clothes: dresses from one hundred to two hundred dollars and trousers starting at fifty dollars; blouses from eighty dollars to $150. I guess retailers figure they have a captive market, so they charge accordingly.

The clothes at this particular boutique are lovely. (Remember the bad old days, when all they offered were prim, blue dresses with a red bow at the neck?) They use very few maternity manufacturers. Instead they use normal designers and ask them to do a maternity version of their usual designs. The clothes here look more realistic than some of the fuddy-duddy designs that maternity designers come up with.

I took Hannah and Laura with me, and they had a blast in the changing room, where there was a nine-month, strap-on stomach. They roared with laughter at my profile and then tried the stomach on themselves. They were leaning up against the wall, overcome with mirth at their pregnant shapes. This is a snooty, upmarket boutique, so I tried to quell the hilarity. I bought a pair of black trousers, cut narrow on the leg, as I like them. I balked at paying fifty-five dollars, but I'll buy only one more maternity outfit. They had some attractive, lace nursing bras in this boutique. I had searched in our local mall, where all the bras were white and looked as if they had been made from huge, flannel sheets. Pregnancy is a time when many women feel large and bulky and unattractive, so if you can find flattering clothes and underwear, it's a psychological boost.

Sunday, November 7

Felt nauseated and dizzy at Mass and had to sit outside in the fresh air. I managed to go back inside for Communion. When I receive Communion now, I am struck by the lines, "Bring us health in mind and body", and now I have two bodies requiring the Lord's attention—mine and his/hers.

By afternoon I was so sick I threw up and felt relief after this. A girlfriend advised me to cut out all vitamins when nauseated. I did this and felt much better on Monday, so shall stay off them until I feel better. Some say no vitamins, some say double the intake of vitamins. I guess we have to experiment to see what works.

WEEK TEN

People who have children and are struggling along on a single income sometimes think of the children as burdens, in the sense that they keep us poor. Many of us have yuppie friends with no kids (DINKS, double income, no kids) or maybe one child who is in permanent day care while both parents bring in a paycheck. While we don't want to put our kids in day care, we envy our friends their financial security.

So I was interested when watching TV last night to see Shelley Winters being interviewed. The actress, now in her seventies, has financial security—a beautiful home in Beverly Hills and an apartment in New York with a view of Central Park and the New York skyline. But Winters has only one child and one grandchild.

"If I have one regret in life," she said, "it is not having had more children and more grandchildren. My grandson is worth more to me than all my money, all my lovers, my three husbands and my Oscar. I consider him the crowning achievement of my life."

It's nice to think that, for someone who has everything materially, children are still the crowning achievement, the only truly worthwhile thing in life. In our hearts we know this, but it's good to remind ourselves occasionally.

I remember being struck by that thought when I was pregnant with Luke, my first baby. It struck me that I was carrying within me someone who would live forever and that no career I could build—as a writer, a lawyer, a doctor—could ever begin to be as important as this child who would exist throughout eternity.

Women who choose to stay home and devote

themselves to raising their kids appreciate the importance of building up the child's character and soul to prepare him to live in eternity with God. What I build as a mother will exist forever.

This does not mean that staying home is always easy, especially if you have had an exciting career in the past. Before I gave birth to Luke, I had enjoyed working as a journalist on newspapers and then doing airline public relations. In the latter career I earned great money (better than my roommate, an attorney), took several overseas trips to write articles and, of course, enjoyed overseas vacations for next to nothing. I remember one overseas flight from Auckland to Los Angeles cost me only twenty-eight dollars.

So, when I had the baby, I was overwhelmed with guilt. I wanted the baby more than any career, more than a million dollars. But I still felt guilty for sitting at home doing nothing but holding the baby. Every week I thought, "Gosh, I could have written two articles and brought in hundreds of dollars this week. Instead, I have done nothing but play with Luke." It was a career woman's guilt. I was equating valuable work with production and paychecks. Not that I *wanted* to be back writing full time. I just felt guilty about not being busy, not producing anything (except a milky breast for Luke) and not helping Ed pay the bills.

That was ten years ago. Today I understand motherhood better. Now I feel zero guilt. I am confident that being an at-home mom is the best career for me. I believe this is where God wants me right now, and I am doing the best I can for my children. Plus, it's fun. I love being at home. I love not having to get into a suit and makeup and drive to work. I love having no boss, no deadlines, no conferences. I understand that some mothers really do have to work, because society is structured for two-income families today. Nevertheless, I am grateful that we can make ends meet on one income. I am grateful that Ed allows me to stay home (even though I have to remind him occasionally that I do *not* lie in the bathtub all day reading novels!).

Week Eleven

Tuesday, November 16

Last week I had a phone call from a young friend who has an eight-month-old baby and is pregnant again. She had developed a breast infection (probably from too infrequent nursing), and the obstetrician had told her (as obstetricians usually do) to stop nursing on the infected side.

This is exactly the information I received nine years ago when nursing Luke, and, after letting my breasts get too full, I got a blocked and infected breast duct. My obstetrician told me the same thing. "Stop nursing immediately."

In fact, this is the worst advice you can receive. I knew from my own experience at the time that the solution was to nurse more frequently than ever on the infected side (on both sides actually) so as to clear the blocked duct and keep the breast empty. Heating pads are also useful. The experts on the breast are not obstetricians but the La Leche League, whose phone numbers are available in any local phone directory. Doctors tell you that if you continue nursing, the baby will catch the infection. But La Leche points out that studies show that the baby is not harmed in any way by continuing to nurse. Antibodies are formed in the milk that protect the baby from the bacteria causing the infection.

The La Leche bible, *The Womanly Art of Breastfeeding* (3d ed., Franklin Park, Ill.: La Leche League, 1981), which every nursing mom should possess, states:

> Sudden weaning is an emotional and physical shock, to both you and the baby, and the breast engorgement that would follow sudden weaning would only make the infection worse. According to a study of many mothers, continued nursing helps clear the infection much faster. An empty breast heals faster and nothing empties the breast so well as your baby's nursing. If your doctor advises you to discontinue breastfeeding, let him know that you feel very strongly about continuing. Your firm convictions may change the doctor's mind. If not, get another opinion from a doctor who is knowledgeable and supportive of breastfeeding (p. 243).

The League says to take antibiotics for the infection, if your doctor prescribes them, but do not stop nursing.

My girlfriend, being in early pregnancy, did not want to take antibiotics and, because she had no fever, just started resting, applying heat and feeding frequently. In forty-eight hours the pain and tenderness were gone.

I cannot recommend La Leche highly enough to young, nursing mothers (or for us old ducks, for that matter!). The women are so kind and helpful when you phone for advice. And for young moms it is worthwhile attending some of their meetings, where you will be surrounded by other moms with babies and toddlers. It is a good way to befriend women who are in the same stage of life as you are. If you can't attend meetings, the La Leche book is fantastic. I referred to it constantly when nursing Luke and will no doubt use it again with this baby, because it will be seven years since I breast fed, and I may be "rusty".

How am I feeling physically at eleven weeks? I am still nauseated and gag occasionally—something I did not suffer from very much in my first three pregnancies. I have cut out the prenatal vitamins altogether, because they are too hard on my stomach right now. I have not gained any weight but am maintaining my usual 145 lbs. I finally have a slightly protruding belly but can still fit into my trousers. I am still sleepy but not as bad as in those first weeks before I knew I was pregnant. I am still waking like clockwork every morning between 2 and 3 A.M. in order to relieve my bladder, but I know this will change as the baby gets bigger and the pressure shifts off my bladder and is more evenly dispersed.

I was thinking about breast-feeding today and what a joy it will be to nurse another baby. I find breast-feeding a "eucharistic" experience—both pregnancy and breast-feeding, actually.

As mothers, we give our bodies to keep the baby alive for nine months. Then after birth, if we nurse totally (i.e., without introducing any supplements or foods) for, say, another four or five months, we become vividly aware that it is still our own bodies that are nourishing the baby. This little creature is growing and thriving simply by feeding on my body.

Breast-feeding made me look at the Eucharist with new eyes. For are we not all his babies? And isn't it his body, blood, soul and divinity that nourish us in the deepest sense? "Unless you eat my body and drink my blood, you can have no life in you. For my body is real food; my blood is real drink" (Jn 6:49–59).

To people outside the Catholic Church, the Eucharist sounds cannibalistic. But seen through the eyes of a nursing mother, it is perfectly comprehensible and beautiful. To give one's body in order to feed the beloved. What could be more natural?

The idea struck me forcibly one morning after I had just given birth to Hannah. A sweet nun brought me Holy Communion. Hannah was on my breast at the time, and Sister said, "Don't bother putting her in the crib. You can receive while holding her." So there

I was, feeding on the body of the Lord while Hannah fed on me.

Thursday, November 18

A girlfriend called me today. "I have a mouthful of chocolate pudding", I told her. "And I have just eaten a whole jar of Mexican salsa."

"You sound like a normal pregnant woman", she said.

We've all heard those stories of pregnant women and their strange "cravings". But a whole jar of salsa? I had never in my life eaten a jar of salsa.

It began yesterday: I was feeling nauseated and threw up at lunchtime. We had been invited to dine with friends, and I was unsure whether I should go. (Incidentally, I have found that chewing gum helps with the queasy feeling. Perhaps it's the fresh, mint taste in your mouth that distracts from the nausea.) Ed talked me into going, and once at our friends' house I started eating chips dipped in salsa. It was so good that for dinner I ate only bread rolls with salsa on them, much to the astonishment of my hostess! Then, driving home at midnight, I made Ed run into the supermarket and buy me a jar of salsa. The next morning I had salsa on toast for breakfast! And kept eating it all day till the jar was empty and I was breathing fire.

I don't call it a craving. I think occasionally pregnant women can't face "normal" food, but then they encounter something that doesn't make them feel queasy, and they are so delighted that they fixate on that particular food, hence the "pickles and ice cream" complex.

WEEK TWELVE

How is the baby doing?

The baby is now about three inches long. His heart is pumping blood that it has formed within itself. He has stumpy little limbs. His eyes are formed. His ears are obvious at the side of the head, and nostrils are appearing on the nose. His brain is sending electrical impulses, and his sex can be identified. He is moving rapidly within the womb, and his movements could be seen on ultrasound, although it is too soon for the mother to feel them. He feels pain or touch stimuli.

I am supposed to have blood tests this week, before my next doctor's appointment, but have decided not to. Next week I am off to New Zealand with the children to visit grandparents and family for three weeks. I donated blood once and felt tired for two weeks, so I shall delay my blood tests till I get back from the trip. I don't want to be tired and anemic when facing hordes of family and in-laws.

Hannah was storming and raging like a spoiled brat today (probably exhausted from another busy day in first grade). I lay down with her in my arms to calm her down, and she fell asleep. Sometimes our children cause us anger and suffering by their behavior, but it's hard not to hold them close.

A single person finds it difficult to understand unconditional love and unconditional forgiveness. But a parent knows. Shakespeare's King Lear said, "How sharper than a serpent's tooth it is to have a thankless child." Yes, our children can cause us pain, but it would not be natural for us to hate them. The normal way we view our children is with hope, patience and prayer.

Having children also helps us appreciate how God can be merciful. Often we wonder how God can forgive us for this sin or that sin. Are we beyond redemption? At those times I think, "Is there anything my child could do that would alienate me from him forever? Is there anything so terrible that his repentance would not soften my heart?" Of course the answer is No, nothing. If my child is sorry, I will always forgive. I can understand the beautiful story of the Prodigal Son. I understand why the father went out every day and looked down the road to see if his brat was coming home.

I find the Divine Mercy devotion of Sister Faustina consoling. Our Lord told Faustina that *trust* is the vessel we must use to draw down his mercy, and so we say each day, "Jesus, I trust in Thee."

Monday, November 22

Had my second visit to the obstetrician today—fairly routine. He checked the size of my uterus, tried to find a heartbeat but said nine weeks from conception was usually too early to hear anything. He asked me again if I wanted to have an amniocentesis. "No, doctor", I told him. "If the baby is Down's syndrome, it will be a well-loved Down's-syndrome child." He smiled, and we left it at that.

Nobody hopes to have an imperfectly formed child. But I read in a life of Saint Gerard Majella that the mother of a blind daughter had begged the saint to restore the child's sight. Majella replied, "If Catherine could see, she would lose her soul."

The story may or may not be true. Nevertheless, is it not possible that God sometimes allows certain of us to be handicapped for our own spiritual good?

On the front page of our local newspaper this week was a picture of a Down's-syndrome teenager competing in the Special Olympics and looking happy and triumphant after winning his swim race. The caption described him as a "special" person. Yes, I thought, once they are born we call them "special", but in the womb they are the victims of clever search-and-destroy techniques, i.e., amniocentesis followed by saline abortions.

If some tests were available to find out if babies were going to be born black or Jewish or homosexual, so that mothers could have the choice to abort—

imagine the outcry! Spokesmen from these populations would cry bloody murder and demand the testing be stopped. But there is no Down's-syndrome spokesman to stand up and demand to know why he and his colleagues are targeted for extinction.

Why do obstetricians push so resolutely for testing? Because of a phenomenon called "wrongful birth" or "wrongful life" suits. In the recent past, a very small number of obstetricians have been sued by women who delivered abnormal babies. The women said that, if the abnormalities had been detected before birth, they would have aborted the babies. The women sued the doctors for not having advised them to have the tests.

These cases are rare. But not long ago a mother in the San Francisco Bay area brought a wrongful life suit against her obstetrician because her baby had been born with spina bifida and was paralyzed from the waist down. The baby also suffered from hydrocephalus. The mother said her obstetrician had failed to give her a test that could have revealed the defects. She said she would have aborted her son if she had been given the choice. Because the test is not offered until between week fifteen and twenty, this would have been a large, well-formed baby whose skull would have required manual crushing after saline poisoning.

One sympathizes with mothers of handicapped infants—raising normal children is hard work, raising a handicapped child must be overwhelmingly difficult.

Nevertheless, one wonders how a child feels, knowing his mother has publicly stated that she wishes she had aborted him. The Lord said about all human beings (Is 43:4), "You are precious in my eyes and I love you." The child confined to a wheelchair is precious in God's eyes.

This explains the motivation of obstetricians in pushing testing on women, but it does not exonerate them morally. The doctor is protecting his bank account, and the pawn in the game is the baby.

My father, in one of his books, suggests that doctors protect themselves by providing patients with a written statement along these lines: "Some physicians would advise amniocentesis or chorionic villus sampling in cases like yours. I do not, because I think it is wrong, dangerous and cruel. But if you wish to have it done, you are at liberty to consult some other obstetrician" (H. P. Dunn, *Ethics for Doctors, Nurses and Patients*, New York: Alba House, 1994, p. 123).

The obstetrician might lose a few patients, but he would probably sleep better at night.

The Second Trimester

Weeks Thirteen, Fourteen and Fifteen

These three weeks were spent with the children in New Zealand, visiting grandparents and family, so you will excuse me if I was not faithful at keeping up my diary. Too much fun, hilarity and rich food!

Do pregnancy and travel mix? New Zealand is seven thousand miles from the west coast of the United States—a gruelling twelve-hour flight on a 747. Add to this the hour-and-twenty-minute flight from San Francisco to Los Angeles to connect with the Air New Zealand 747, plus the two-hour wait at LAX airport, and it adds up to a long, tiring journey. Plus, I was travelling without Ed. So, how does the pregnant body hold up?

My doctor's only advice was to take extra fluids on board the aircraft, because the cabin is dehydrating, and to exercise the legs by walking up and down the aisles occasionally, to prevent ankle swelling. I ignored his advice on toting extra fluids because, between the luggage and Barbie dolls, teddy bears and coats, I knew I could not cope with carrying anything else. Besides, the planes are stocked with plenty of drinks. I sipped orange juice and tomato juice on the flight and did not feel dehydrated.

I had read in a book about a seven-months pregnant woman, flying to Brazil, who said her ankles were the size of footballs by the time she arrived, so I kept mine raised as much as possible. Usually, this meant tucking them into the seat pocket in front of me. Anything is better than having them flat on the floor, where the blood collects around the ankles. I had no swelling on either this flight or the return flight, although I suspect if I had been more advanced in pregnancy I might have had some.

The only unpleasant experience I had was gagging as I walked through LAX after the return flight. Although not generally nauseated now, I find if I get overly tired or stressed, I start retching. On this flight back to California, I had been awake and active for twenty-five hours by the time we reached Los Angeles. I felt nauseated and dizzy. (Southern California is generally regarded as the home of some looney toons, so the sight of a woman gagging en route from one plane to another didn't elicit much attention. Onlookers probably thought I'd been smoking weed!) It was wonderful to see Ed again and be smothered in his bear hug. But Luke was ill that first night home, so I got very little sleep watching him during the night. By the following morning, I was totally wasted. It took a week to recover fully from jet lag.

While in New Zealand, I made it a point not to go out at night. I did all my visiting during the day, then retired by 9 P.M. or 10 P.M. and slept late. This made for an enjoyable, stress-free visit. My mom spoiled me rotten and did all the cooking and dishes while I was

WEEKS THIRTEEN TO FIFTEEN 57

there. Aren't mothers wonderful? Mine is seventy-six, has had seven children (the seventh at age forty-five) and still has the energy to spoil me. Some women speak negatively of being "worn out by childbearing", but when I look at women of my mom's generation who are strong and fit and enjoying life after raising large families, it undermines that claim. Childbearing seems to foster strength in these women.

Perhaps, while on the subject of "Downunder", it's a good opportunity to say a little about IVF, seeing that Australia used to lead the world in this technology.

IVF, or in-vitro fertilization (fertilization outside the womb, often popularly called test-tube reproduction), is so accepted today that I personally know three women who have undergone the procedure, and, after huge expense and numerous miscarriages, two produced babies. The third gave up and accepted her infertility.

The IVF procedure produces numerous "leftover" embryos, which are either frozen or discarded. One of these mothers told me she left the embryos with the doctor and told him, "Do what you like with them." She had no further interest in the fate of her offspring.

In the United States we have seen legal battles over the fate of these leftover embryos: In the case of divorce, who owns them? Can the divorced wife be implanted with some embryos against her divorced husband's wishes? Do the embryos have the right to inherit if there are no living children when spouses die? The legal battles are bizarre, but then so is the whole IVF procedure.

In his 1994 "Letter to Families", Pope John Paul II said that what is acceptable with animals is not acceptable in human reproduction. About fourteen years ago, when I was a young, unmarried reporter, I did a story on some doctors in Melbourne, Australia, who were leading the world in IVF at that stage. I vividly remember that on the door of the doctor's clinic hung a sign, "We pay ten dollars for sperm samples." I wondered how many foolish men were seduced by the ten-dollar fee to produce sperm by masturbation and then had no interest in where their sperm were used. Obviously, the sperm were being used by women trying to achieve conception, and these sperm donors were becoming fathers of children they would never meet or know—all for a paltry ten dollars. It reduced human sexuality to the level of breeding cattle.

IVF is the separation of procreation from sex, and, as such, it is the flip side of contraception, which is the separation of sex from procreation. The Church opposes IVF because procreation must be limited to the loving sexual embrace of husband and wife. Also, the Church teaches that the genetic material exchanged in a marriage should be that of the husband and wife, not of a third party, as happens when a sperm donor or donated egg is introduced into the equation. This amounts to technological adultery.

IVF is barbaric in other ways: women undergoing

the procedure must agree to have an abortion if abnormality is suspected in the fetus. Furthermore, because of overstimulation of the ovaries, the mother often has a multiple pregnancy. Then, in order to reduce the number of babies to ensure survival of one or two, the doctor uses a new technique, called "selective reduction of pregnancies", to eliminate two or three babies. This is done at around the twenty-week stage. The doctor pierces the unwanted babies through the heart with a long needle attached to a syringe and injects potassium chloride, which stops the heart from beating.

Does this sound farfetched? In a 1990 article in the medical magazine *Lancet,* Dr. R. J. Wapner reported that he and seven colleagues had managed forty-six pregnancies this way in a Philadelphia hospital. There were about 230 babies at the beginning, and they were reduced to seventy-five live babies—all through injections into the heart. One wonders about these obstetricians and what their fate will be when they finally stand before God's throne. Will thousands of their victim fetuses rise up to demand justice? What judgment will await medical geniuses who exterminate these little ones who have no voice and no strength to fight back?

Often when we see those cute pictures of yet another test-tube baby snuggled in mom's arms, we are unmindful of all the immoral acts that lead up to an IVF birth: the masturbation, the introduction of a third-party egg or sperm (in some cases, though often these are from the spouses), the freezing or discarding of leftover live embryos who have immortal souls but no womb to bring them to birth, the agreement by the mother to abort defective fetuses and the use of the "selective reduction technique" to abort multiple fetuses. All in all, IVF is not a pretty picture, although the poor baby in the photograph is innocent of his origins.

The best book I have read on the new reproductive technologies is *Infertility—Women Speak Out about Their Experiences of Reproductive Medicine*, edited by Renate D. Klein (London, Sydney, Wellington: Pandora Press, 1989; unavailable in the United States but could be ordered through an American book store). Strangely enough, of the forty women from many countries who contribute to the book, most are feminists. Yet the women are disgusted at how the new technologies treat women. The book alleges that the media have glamorized IVF and that doctors at IVF clinics lie to women when they say IVF is highly successful. Doctors brag about the high conception rate but do not go on to explain that there is also an extremely high miscarriage rate. (The three women I know all experienced multiple miscarriages.) Only a small percentage of women (5 percent to 10 percent) actually produce a live baby. Klein's book calls IVF "a failed technology", which uses women as "living test sites" for drugs and dangerous techniques.

The book includes stories of women who have died

from having their ovaries overstimulated by fertility hormones—usually clomid or pergonal. As many as forty-seven eggs have been collected at one time from one woman, whereas in a normal cycle a woman releases only one or occasionally two eggs. Other health problems the book details include ovarian cysts, septicemia, migraines, dizziness, vision problems, weight gain and depression, breast and ovarian cancer. Klein asks why women are not warned of the huge risk of IVF treatment.

One example is that of Rivi Ben Ari, of Israel, who died suddenly while being treated with pergonal to stimulate her ovaries for egg collection. The pergonal caused her blood to clot so thickly it could not be tested, because it clotted in the syringe. Ultrasound showed many large cysts on her ovaries and an accumulation of fluids caused by the overstimulation. She was finally diagnosed with edema (swelling) in the brain. She was declared brain dead, and twenty-four hours later she was clinically dead.

Klein's book also points out the health problems of babies born of IVF—the high number of cesarean sections, premature births and babies with low birth weight, as well as a greater chance of having a baby with spina bifida or cardiac problems.

The Catholic Church has spoken out against these reproductive technologies, but the average layman seems to know little about the immorality of the techniques used or the health hazards.

I am getting off the subject of my pregnancy, so let's

just end with a quote from *Donum Vitae* (The Gift of Life), the Instruction from the Congregation for the Doctrine of the Faith on "Respect for Human Life in Its Origins and on the Dignity of Procreation. Replies to Certain Questions of the Day". The document (which bears Cardinal Ratzinger's signature) states in part:

> The connection between in vitro fertilization and the voluntary destruction of human embryos occurs too often. This is significant: through these procedures, with apparently contrary purposes, life and death are subjected to the decision of man, who thus sets himself up as the giver of life and death by decree. This dynamic of violence and domination may remain unnoticed by those very individuals who, in wishing to utilize this procedure, become subject to it themselves. The facts recorded and the cold logic that links them must be taken into consideration for a moral judgment on IVF and ET (in vitro fertilization and embryo transfer): the abortion mentality which has made this procedure possible thus leads, whether one wants it or not, to man's domination over the life and death of his fellow human beings and can lead to a system of radical eugenics (Part II, para. 3).

Week Sixteen

Tuesday, December 21

I have now gained five pounds and am showing a little. Today I had a blood test, and the nurse told me they are checking for anemia, immunity to rubella, syphilis and hepatitis. Hepatitis would also be an indicator of whether a person had AIDS, although she said they are not specifically testing for AIDS.

I think they should test for AIDS as a protection for the doctor and for the mother's own information. But homosexual groups have been politically successful in making mandatory AIDS testing a sensitive issue. Many women have already been tested (as I was) when they took out life insurance.

One of the main benefits of testing would be to protect the unborn baby. In 1994 the National Institute of Allergy and Infectious Diseases released the results of a study (called ACTG 076) that was reported in *Drug Topics* (July 25, 1994) 138:29. This study involved 477 HIV positive pregnant women who were treated either with the drug AZT or a placebo during pregnancy. Their babies were then given the drug during the first six weeks of life. Results showed that HIV transmission to the baby was reduced by two thirds in the women treated with AZT (as compared to the placebo group), lowering the transmission rate to 8.3 percent.

A similar study, whose lead author was Pamela Boyer, M.D., Ph.D., of the Department of Obstetrics and Gynecology at UCLA School of Medicine, found that HIV transmission to unborn babies was reduced to 4 percent when AZT was administered to the mothers. Interestingly, this study did not treat the infants with AZT for six weeks after birth, which raises the question of whether the infants need to be treated at all.

Another reason for pregnant women to get tested is to prevent their passing the HIV virus to their babies through breast-feeding, as the virus is present in breast milk. I would suggest testing for any pregnant woman who might have been exposed to AIDS through sex, blood transfusion or caring for AIDS patients.

Why do I mention those who might have been caring for AIDS patients? Although the media downplay the risks of casual infection with HIV, Stanley Monteith, M.D., in his book *AIDS: the Unnecessary Epidemic* (Sevierville, Tenn.: Covenant House Books, 1991), discusses the famous "Splash Cases", which even the media were forced to report on back in 1987. These were the three female health-care workers who were infected as a result of blood coming in contact with their *intact* skin. One woman got a small spot of blood on her finger and had it there for twenty minutes before washing her hands. The second woman was drawing blood from a patient when the top of a tube flew off and blood splattered into her mouth and on her face. The third woman spilled blood onto her face and hands from a machine that separated blood components. Dr. Monteith describes how all three women were found to be HIV positive in a matter of months after being splashed with infected blood. Monteith writes, "Thus by May of 1987 physicians recognized that infected blood on a person's skin could lead to a fatal infection" (p. 188). This, however, is not something that is stressed in the media.

A word here about diet and exercise—a word that might get me into trouble, but I must be honest. Often, pregnant women become very virtuous about diet and exercise. This is especially true of American women, I have noticed, but less true of Australian and New Zealand women, probably because of the more relaxed attitude of doctors in those countries. I must confess to being a slug. I am a slug when nonpregnant and a slug when pregnant. I do not jog, lift weights or swim lengths. I have never watched an exercise video in my life. In spite of this, I consider myself to be of average weight for my height and fairly fit . . . as slugs go. When pregnant, I continue as normal and do not feel disadvantaged because I have not donned leotards, tap-danced or jogged. I eat as I normally would, except that I try to eliminate junk food, and I am careful about taking vitamins. I keep a closer eye on my weight because I know how easy it is for pregnancy to be an excuse to pig out, and I do not want to carry extra pounds. The thirty allowable pounds are more than enough for my legs.

My worst sin when pregnant is that I occasionally (and I stress *occasionally*) allow myself a glass of wine with dinner. I realize this goes against doctor's orders, but I am confident this moderate intake (all things in moderation) does not harm the baby.

I think some pregnant women go overboard on exercise and cutting out all alcohol and caffeine in order to produce the perfect baby. This is fine if you have one or two children but, if you had ten children, imagine going seven and a half pregnant years (90 months) living on apple juice, lettuce leaves, de-caffeinated tea and other virtuous foods. Pregnancy is hard work. I think women deserve an occasional treat, like a cup of tea and a chocolate cookie. (However, I stress that this is a personal opinion, and I am not advocating that women disregard doctor's orders. If you are the type who cannot stop at one glass of wine a week or one cup of coffee, then I'd say don't indulge at all.)

I asked my younger sister, who lives in Venice, Italy, whether the Italian doctors allow a pregnant woman to have a sip of wine occasionally.

"Oh sure", Liz said. "Italian doctors are very laid back. They're a law unto themselves. Mine sits at his desk, smoking like a chimney, and tells me between hacking coughs, 'You need to take better care of your health!' "

Week Seventeen

How is the baby doing?

The baby now measures nine inches in length and weighs about six ounces. There is fine lanugo hair on his head. His fingernails are perfectly formed. He has eyelids that he can open and close, although they usually remain closed at this stage. Soon I hope to feel the baby move, as it is between weeks sixteen and twenty that mom becomes aware of movement. As well as moving his arms and legs vigorously, the baby can wiggle his toes and perform little "kissing" movements with his mouth. The baby is drinking the amniotic fluid, which also flows in and out of the baby's lungs. (This does not drown the baby, because he is not yet dependent on his lungs for oxygen. The oxygen is provided by mother through the oxygenated blood of the placenta.)

Monday, December 27

Today I heard the heart beat! Last visit the doctor had tried to detect it, but it was too faint for his Doppler. This time, as soon as he put the instrument on my abdomen, there was a loud, steady heartbeat. My eyes widened. Even though this is my fourth baby, it is still surprising to hear someone else's heart beating within me; to know that I really do have a living being within. The kids (who are off school for Christmas vacation) and I went out to lunch to celebrate the heartbeat.

One thing during this visit disappointed me. I had written to my insurance company to ask them if they would pick up the cost of my getting a midwife or nurse practitioner to assist me as a coach during my labor. I had one for my second pregnancy, and I credit her with helping me have such a wonderful vaginal birth experience after having had a cesarean for my first baby.

In fact, I had been reading the book *How to Avoid a Cesarean Section*, by Christopher Norwood (New York: Simon and Schuster, 1984), which strongly recommends that women trying to achieve a VBAC (vaginal birth after cesarean) get a labor coach. Norwood writes:

> For women . . . who aren't satisfied with the cesarean rate of the available facilities [in their communities] or who simply want their labor to be as tranquil as possible—there is an option. Consider hiring an obstetric nurse or other trained "labor support" person to stay with you at home through the start of labor and then accompany you to the hospital.
>
> Often, childbirth activist groups which have screened local doctors will also have a list of obstetric nurses or childbirth educators who are happy to go to a woman's home and then to the hospital and coach her individually. It is hard to exaggerate the real enthusiasm and interest these nurses and coaches

bring to labor. You will go through the birth process with a professional who is on your side. Also, a nurse can measure your progress—even a female obstetrician in labor cannot tell by herself how far she is dilated—and prevent you from going to the hospital too soon, where "protocol" may begin to take over (p. 102).

I would add that, even for women who have never had a cesarean, a labor coach who can check dilatation at home is a big plus and will help any woman avoid unnecessary surgery.

One interesting point in Norwood's book was this:

> In a provocative insight into the conditions of normal delivery, McMaster University Medical Center in Ontario, Canada, has reported that, no matter what a mother's reason for a previous cesarean, if she arrived at the hospital more than 3 centimeters dilated, she had a 67 percent chance of having a normal delivery—with less than 3 centimeters dilation, the chances were much smaller (p. 121).

I find this easy to believe. It is better to have a coach tell you "Go to the hospital now. You are in good labor." Because if you go when not in good labor, you will likely be strapped to a hospital bed, tied to a fetal monitor, perhaps have a drip thrust in your arm, and it is difficult to labor under those conditions. Then, when the hospital gets bored with you, you run the risk of having a cesarean.

Anyway . . . what disappointed me during this visit

was that my insurance company said I could have a nurse practitioner to coach me, but my obstetrician said No. I get the impression that he is paranoid about being sued. He said he would not be "held responsible" if the coach did not get me to the hospital on time and I had the baby in the car. Needless to say, if this happened, of course I would not hold him responsible. Still, his attitude left me wondering if he was the right obstetrician for me after all.

Then another strange thing happened, which filled me with doubt about my obstetrician. When I first went to see him, I was given a letter stating (and I quote exactly), "Your insurance requires you to have one screening ultrasound at approximately 18 weeks." Now, I have nothing against ultrasound, which is a useful screening tool. However, not all the information is in on the complete safety of ultrasound, which uses sound waves to bring the baby's image up on a screen for viewing. General consensus is that it is safer than X ray, but it may take a few more generations to know fully what effects it has on the baby. Therefore, I am not keen on routine ultrasound. But I don't mind having one if the doctor thinks the baby is not growing or there is some other problem.

Although in Britain the Royal College of Obstetricians and Gynecologists has accepted a policy of routine scanning at sixteen weeks, the American College of Obstetricians and Gynecologists takes a different view. This college says, "No well-controlled study has yet proved that routine scanning of all prenatal patients will improve the outcome of pregnancy" and recommends that "at present, only indicated diagnostic studies should be ordered." Similarly, the U.S. Department of Health and Human Services has written: "Ultrasound should be limited to situations in which there is an accepted medical reason for the procedure. . . . There is not enough evidence that routine screening benefits either the mother or the fetus."

An article in the *Wall Street Journal* (Oct. 8, 1993, part A, page 5A) describes how Australian researchers have found that frequent ultrasound examinations during pregnancy may restrict fetal growth. Researchers at King Edward Memorial Hospital in Perth, Australia, studied 2,834 women. Half were given just one ultrasound test during the eighteenth week of pregnancy, while the rest underwent five or more tests between weeks eighteen and thirty-eight. The babies in this latter group were more than twice as likely to have a low birth weight. This seems to indicate that, while one test during pregnancy might be harmless, repeated tests might not be.

An article in the *New England Journal of Medicine* (Sept. 16, 1993, 329:874) described a 1984 study by the National Institutes of Health that found no evidence that ultrasound reduced perinatal disease or mortality. The article reported, "A 1993 study that screened more than 15,000 low-risk pregnant women with ultrasound confirmed this." However, the article suggests that women in high-risk pregnancies may well benefit from ultrasound screenings.

I also found an FDA warning (*FDA Consumer*, Sept. 1995, 29:31) advising companies that perform ultrasounds on pregnant women not to make videos of the unborn babies, because the videos were not medically necessary and might potentially harm the fetus. I understand there is a growing trend for women to want take-home videos of the baby's antics in the womb. One doctor told me that he doesn't recommend routine ultrasounds but women pressure him because they think having an ultrasound is fun and they want a photo of the baby.

Not long ago, I was reading one of Sheila Kitzinger's books (*The Complete Book of Pregnancy and Childbirth* [New York: Knopf, 1989]), and this is what she writes on the subject:

> Although ultrasound has not been proven safe, it is probably much safer than x-rays, which provided the only method of finding out about the baby in the uterus before the scan was developed. High frequency sounds continued for a long time can cause damage to the hearing in an adult. Questions have therefore been raised about possible effects on the baby's hearing, since although the sound waves are only bounced off the baby for a short time, the baby may be vulnerable at certain stages of its development. Babies are not born deaf after having ultrasound, but no one yet knows if any of them will suffer delayed effects in later life (p. 204).

This interested me because my firstborn, Luke, is the only baby I permitted to have the ultrasound (at twelve-weeks gestation), and he is the only one of the three who has significant ear problems. He has had two sets of tubes for ear infections, and his hearing is not as good as that of the other two. I believe there is an increase in ear infections in today's youngsters. It makes one wonder if the increase might be connected in any way to the millions of routine ultrasounds performed today. . . .

I called the insurance company to ask if there was any way I could be excused from the "required" ultrasound.

"We don't require an ultrasound. How could we? We are not doctors", the insurance spokesman told me. He added, "It's probably just the way your doctor words it so he doesn't have to justify the ultrasound."

I was amazed to hear this and called my obstetrician. "My insurance company says they don't 'require' an ultrasound, and I'd prefer not to have one unless indicated", I said.

"Okay, fine", was all he said.

I never did push the issue of why he had pretended it was an insurance requirement. By now I was feeling negative vibes about my doctor. I got the impression that his main thrust was to protect himself from lawsuits rather than to help the woman have a healthy, comfortable pregnancy and delivery. After discussion with my husband, I decided to try to find another obstetrician.

Saturday, January 1, 1994

On New Year's Day, at the end of week seventeen, I felt a slight flutter in my lower abdomen. Could this be the baby moving?

The next day, movements were definitely detectable. This palpable movement—quickening is the old-fashioned term, from the saying "The quick and the dead"—is exciting and reassuring. Of course, the baby has been moving actively for about six weeks now but not strongly enough to be felt by mom. When I placed my fingers on my lower abdomen, while lying in bed, I could feel a gentle fluttering.

WEEK EIGHTEEN

Wednesday, January 5

This week I received permission from my insurance company to change doctors. I have found a doctor who lives closer to me and who is in practice with a midwife who has a great reputation for helping women to have normal (i.e., nonsurgical) deliveries. As opposed to my former doctor, this doctor will

— turn a breech baby, even with a woman who has had a previous cesarean;

— turn a breech even during labor;

— use forceps to assist the mother if required; and

— allow me to have a midwife as my labor coach both at home and in the delivery room.

I have not yet been to visit him, but I feel already that with this obstetrician I will be more comfortable that he is going to let me try for a normal delivery.

I have now gained eight pounds and am definitely showing—even wearing a nursing bra, as my old bras are too tight.

Week Nineteen

Monday, January 10

I had a brief meeting with my new doctor. He is definitely more laid back than the other one. (He even agreed that a glass of wine with dinner was fine!) With a New York accent and untidily knotted necktie, he leaned back in his office chair and reassured me that he had no problems with turning a breech baby or using forceps in order to avoid a cesarean. An older man in his mid-sixties, he was trained in the days when these procedures were considered normal.

"Americans have gotten sue-crazy, and obstetrics has gotten very technical. I preferred practicing in the old days, when you could relax and play with the baby after delivering it. Now it is whisked away for a battery of tests. It's all very high pressure", he said.

This doctor recently helped a patient have a vaginal delivery after she had had three prior cesareans (not by him). She delivered successfully and was thrilled finally to have had a normal birth.

He approves of having a labor coach, and, in fact, he gave me an article, "The Doula in America: Studying Effects of Support in Labor", by John H. Kennell, M.D. It reads in part:

> In all but one of 150 cultures studied by anthropologists, a family member or friend, usually a woman, remained with a mother during labor and delivery. Before childbirth moved from the home to the hospital in the 20th century, it was also the practice in industrialized nations for family members to support the mother actively in labor, often with the assistance of a trained or untrained midwife. Although more fathers, relatives and friends have been allowed into labor and delivery rooms in the past 20 years, a considerable number of mothers still undergo labor and delivery without the presence of family or close friends.
>
> Since continuous social support during labor is a component of care in a majority of societies but an inconsistent obstetrical practice in our culture, we systematically studied its clinical effect during labor on maternal and neonatal morbidity in an obstetric setting in Guatemala in which mothers routinely undergo labor alone. This social support was pro-

vided by women companions. We enrolled healthy primagravidous mothers using a randomized design. Compared to 249 women laboring alone, 168 mothers with supportive female companions throughout labor had significantly fewer perinatal complications, less need for pitocin augmentation (2.4 vs. 13.3%) and a significantly shorter length of labor (7.7 hours vs. 15.5 hours). The incidence of cesarian sections was also significantly reduced (6.5 versus 17.3%). In addition, fewer infants were admitted to neonatal intensive care.

Kenning says his findings suggest an association between acute anxiety and arrest of labor and fetal distress.

Readers who have had a prior cesarean and would like to attempt normal delivery with the help of a childbirth assistant should write to their insurance companies requesting that they cover this service. Most insurance companies find the $350 fee easier to swallow than the thousands of dollars involved in surgery and a prolonged hospital stay. (I think having my first baby by cesarean cost about $10,000 total—80 percent of which was paid by the insurance company.) Blue Cross picked up my first childbirth assistant, and Aetna has agreed to pick up the fee for this coach.

Week Twenty

Tuesday, January 18

My breasts have developed a life of their own! At three months I had to change from my 38-B bra to my old nursing bras in a 38 C. Then this week I had some breast tenderness and realized that my bra was too tight and was biting into me. So I went to the mall and came home wearing a monstrosity from Mothercare in a size 40 D! Ed says I look like Madonna. (To me, that's the ultimate insult.) I just hope they reduce to their old size after the baby is weaned.

In my previous pregnancies I never noticed my breasts getting large. In fact, it was not till the milk came in a couple of days after birth that they became engorged, so I have no idea why they are swelling up in this pregnancy. They say every pregnancy is different. But I should thank God that I feel fit and healthy as I approach the fifth month. A girlfriend who is seven weeks ahead of me is occasionally bedridden because her pelvic joints are reacting to the weight of the baby by aching so badly that she cannot walk because of the pain. She has to use a wheelchair. This is her sixth pregnancy. When I see what my friend is going through, I am relieved that so far my only problem is that I resemble Dolly Parton.

A pregnant woman is the butt of other people's advice—sometimes unwanted advice. When I was three months along and hadn't gained any weight, a mom told me, "That's bad. You should have gained five pounds by now." When I was four months and had gained three pounds, someone else said, "Three pounds already! You shouldn't have gained that much yet." In a first pregnancy this sort of advice can worry a mom, but because this is my fourth, I don't take much notice of these comments.

As I mentioned earlier, people are full of advice about pregnancy nausea, too, often assuring you that, if you feel sick, your pregnancy is progressing well. But a girlfriend lost her baby at sixteen weeks, and she had thrown up the entire time! The point is that a lot of advice you receive is not worth a dime. As long as you don't let it upset you, it's part of the fun of being pregnant.

You also get the negative comments. "Is this going to be your last?" is a frequent question asked of any woman who dares to have more than two babies.

"No, this is our fourth. We have six more on order", I reply.

I read a funny article once by Gerard and Rita Joseph, parents of eight. When faced with this kind of negative interrogation, Joseph wrote some responses. For example:

> "How many kids do you have?"
> "Eight."
> "Eight! Does your wife work?"
> "No, she broke down a while back, and I haven't had her fixed yet."

"What, another one?"
"No, actually we're recycling the first one."

"Are you going to call it quits now?"
"Well, we were going to call it Stephen if it's a boy."

In our Planned Parenthood dominated society, there is a new form of puritanism, which regards reproduction as an immoral activity. The strange thing is that most of these interrogators have two children whom they would describe as their greatest, most treasured possessions. Yet, if you asked if they would like one more child, they would respond, "No way! Are you crazy?" Scripture regards children as blessings, but Planned Parenthood has been singularly successful in selling the concept that children are a curse . . . unless produced in limited quantities.

Children's attitudes to pregnancy are revealing. I find that in families where the parents may be sterilized, the children who visit our house say negative things about my pregnancy. "Oooh, yuk. We don't want any more babies. We've got enough", they say. Or "I don't like babies. They're too much work. They cost too much money." It is obvious that the children are repeating their parents' attitudes.

This probably explains the spate of children's books in this country that try to justify a new baby to existing siblings. My six-year-old brought one home from the school library recently—all about a three-year-old's negative, hostile feelings toward her newborn brother.

"This is a stupid book", I told Hannah. "Normal children do not hate their baby brothers."

"I know. I'm excited that we're having a baby", she said.

And her reaction is echoed by the children in all the Christian families I know who like babies and are open to having more. These children are always excited when their moms get pregnant. Babies are fun. You have only to look at a baby with its fat cheeks, chicken-feathers hair and hungry, suckling mouth to appreciate that it is beautiful and good. It's a shame that some children are being conditioned to dislike babies.

Friends of ours even took their firstborn to "sibling class" at a local hospital. The class is supposed to ready the existing child for the intrusion of a new sibling. Ed and I were amazed that this couple thought it necessary to have "experts" try to adjust their child's psychology so that he would welcome the new baby.

Back in the dark ages when babies were considered a blessing, was all this negativity present in children? I doubt it. I suspect it is a phenomenon unknown in past generations.

I was surprised when a friend gave me another reason why I shouldn't be having a baby at forty-two.

"Do you realize", my friend asked, "that you'll never have an empty house now?"

"That's great", I replied. "An empty house is not one of my priorities in life."

The interesting thing about this woman is that she

was recently widowed at age forty-five. She has two daughters who are married and living away from home, and she has a nine-year-old son. The son, she once told me, was an unwanted pregnancy, conceived while she was wearing an IUD (intrauterine device). Yet today, especially in the wake of her husband's death, she is the first to admit that it is this nine year old who has given her a reason to live. Without him, she would indeed have "an empty house", and her loneliness would be more intense than it already is.

My youngest sister, Liz, was born when my dad was forty-six (my mom was forty-five), and I remember him saying, "I am the only sixty-year-old on the block with a house full of beautiful, fifteen-year-old girls." My parents said that Liz kept them young. They were up on the latest music and fads because of her. They weren't pining for an empty house; they were happy to have one that resounded with the laughter of youth. I think this is a positive attitude toward late-in-life pregnancy. I might add that Liz is the best looking of us seven children, so perhaps an "old egg" is more glamorous than a "young egg", in spite of doctors' dire predictions.

The bottom line is that we are not producing children just because we want to populate our house. As Christians, we also want to populate heaven with our children. Where the baby is going to be living in twenty years is a shortsighted view. It's where the baby will be living for eternity that's important. As parents, we hope that this child will gain heaven. When I was longing to be pregnant and failing, I kept asking God, "Isn't there room for one more heir to your kingdom?" And, please God, that is the destiny of this little one I am carrying.

WEEK TWENTY-ONE

How is the baby doing?

The fifth month is the "fattening-up month" for the baby—the month when he starts to put on some real weight. He now measures about twelve inches and weighs around fourteen ounces. The doctor can now feel the various parts of the baby's body through the mother's abdomen and tell exactly where the head is and where the buttocks are. At this stage the baby can hiccup, and he may be startled by loud noises. He has definite sleeping and waking phases. Finger- and toenails have started to harden and are very distinct. His bones are becoming stronger and more rigid. His skin is secreting vernix, a white, pasty substance that protects his growing skin from amniotic fluid.

Tuesday, January 25

I had a scare today with my heart. For several days I had felt an unaccustomed fluttering in my heart. It would beat normally and then occasionally give a flutter or palpitation. I called the doctor after the third day but caught him just as the office was closing, and he said as long as I could take deep breaths and was not feeling dizzy, not to worry.

Ed was away in New Zealand for his sister's wedding, so I was a bit unnerved when, that night, at 8 P.M., my heart started again with the wild fluttering about three times every minute. "I can't have a heart attack with three little kids who are too dopey to dial 911", I thought. So I called the local emergency room and asked if I could come in and have a doctor listen to my heart. They said sure, they were not busy.

When I drove in with the kids, they hooked me up to the electrocardiogram. "You're having p.v.c.s (premature ventricular contractions)", the doctor told me. "It is probably due to the extra stress of the pregnancy on your heart. Plus the fact that you are an older mom. A lot of people get them. They are generally harmless, so don't worry about them unless you get shortness of breath, dizziness or chest pains." The doctor advised that I cut out all caffeine and chocolate, which I have since done. (See how one's sins catch up to one?) I am still getting them, but less frequently.

I had my first physical exam and check-up with my new obstetrician. He is reassuring. His cesarean rate is 11 percent, which compares favorably with the national rate of 20 to 25 percent.

The children are so excited about the pending arrival of the baby. The other night, the baby was having a kicking session, so I called Laura in to place her fingers on my lower abdomen. She was rewarded with a sizable kick, which left her grinning from ear to ear.

Thursday, January 27

Ed got home safely from New Zealand last night. I was so happy to see his handsome, sweet face coming down the concourse at the San Francisco airport that I cried when I hugged him. I hadn't realized I missed him so much!

Unfortunately, when he got to work this morning, he found the entire construction company is folding, and he is receiving pay only for the next five days. We were unemployed four months back, so it is less of a shock this time around, and Ed is good at his job (estimating and project management), so I'm sure he will find something else with another company. At times like these, we are thrown back on trust in divine providence.

But it brought to mind what a newly married couple in their thirties told me recently. They were talking about when they would consider getting pregnant, and the husband said, "Not for a couple of years. We have some bills to pay off." I chuckled because most parents would agree that, if we waited till the bills were paid off and we had money in the bank, we would all be childless. I don't think there is ever a financially good time to get pregnant. Sometimes it takes a generous, philosophical husband to accommodate the pregnancy amid the financial disasters of life.

WEEK TWENTY-TWO

Monday, January 31

This week I overdid it and suffered the consequences. So many people have been good to us and showed us hospitality that we had planned to have a party to repay them. Then, when Ed lost the job, we scaled down to a dinner party for ten on Friday night. It was great fun but a lot of work, what with scrubbing floors, tidying my tornado-strewn house, cooking a big roast dinner and then serving it. Some friends stayed till midnight, and I spent a lot of time on my feet, chatting. Then Saturday was a hectic day, helping Ed strip the walls in our master bathroom where the wallpaper had been peeling off.

By Saturday night my pelvic muscles in the groin area were aching so badly I had to go to bed. I could get up only in short bursts to get the kids to brush their teeth and to tuck them in. Sunday morning when I arose, it felt a bit better, but after two hours on my feet the pain was back. The ache was so bad I didn't even go to church. I just lay on my back all day. I had visions of ending up in a wheelchair, the way my girlfriend had.

According to one book, the round ligaments that support the uterus are pulled and stretched at this stage of pregnancy. This causes aches and pains especially between weeks eighteen to twenty-four. One obstetrician refers to this as "pelvic arthropathy", caused by the pelvic joints becoming loose and lax in order to facilitate expansion of the pelvic cavity to allow the baby's head to pass through. This doctor says he has seen women forced to use crutches or be confined to bed if the pain is too great.

Fortunately, by Monday the condition was improved, with only slight twinges in the groin area. To use a layman's description: it feels as though the baby's head is lying right there on the pelvic bone. Or, as one mother put it: it feels as though I've been riding a horse through the desert for a week.

Anyway, the experience taught me not to overdo it. I love to be active, and I have rejoiced in good health up to this five-month stage, but I have to remember that I am forty-two next month and that my aged body needs cosseting if it is to carry this baby safely to term.

Week Twenty-Three

Monday, February 7

I was lying in the bath this evening, thinking, "The kids have strep throat, Luke broke his finger playing football, Ed is unemployed, it's pouring rain, I'm pregnant and I've never been happier."

Even I was amazed at the thought, but it shows how much joy a new life brings. If it were not for the pregnancy, I would regard this winter as a trial, what with unemployment and the usual winter sicknesses, but nothing can spoil our excitement.

I have gained twelve pounds and feel huge, although friends tell me I don't look big, probably because I carry my babies high up under the bustline.

I took Hannah for a brief outing to the mall with me. Sometimes, as a treat, I take one child, so I can relate one-on-one without the others interrupting. There was a light drizzle as we drove. "Rainy days are bad days for ants", Hannah mused.

Later she said, "I wish I had lived when Noah did."

"Why, darling?" I asked.

"Because after the flood it would have been so relaxing with no people around."

Yes, it must have been relaxing, but I hope she is not turning into a population pessimist like Al Gore and Paul Erlich!

Week Twenty-Four

Friday, February 18

This week I discover I have a large varicose vein at the inside top of my thigh. I am sure this developed as a result of my overdoing it the previous weekend and getting the aching groin. My doctor says it is due to the pressure of the baby's weight. He says it will shrink after the baby's birth but not go away completely. Apparently, the small, red spider veins women get on their legs disappear completely after birth, but the varicose veins tend to stay put. I am lucky I have never experienced varicose veins until this fourth pregnancy. But it's a great excuse to put my legs up more often!

I have been thumbing through pregnancy manuals at the local bookstore and am surprised at how much attention is given to sexual intercourse during pregnancy, often in graphic bad taste.

I was appalled at the graphic illustrations of different positions for the sexual act that might prove useful during pregnancy. I wondered how many small children thumb through their mom's pregnancy books looking for pictures of sweet little babies only to find these illustrations.

Most of the manuals speak of "your partner" as opposed to "your husband" and suggest mutual masturbation as an alternative to normal intercourse during pregnancy. This is offensive to Christian readers who consider this behavior morally unacceptable. It strikes me that any husband and wife with half a brain can figure out for themselves how to have normal intercourse without causing discomfort to either mother or baby. We don't require chapter after chapter of sex manual inserted into a pregnancy book, complete with graphic details.

Week Twenty-Five

Monday, February 21

I have dyed my hair red, and Ed is not impressed. "You always dye your hair red when you're pregnant", he complains. He's right. I get tired of looking at my stomach and then tired of my swollen face and decide it would be fun to be someone else. Fortunately, it is one of those dyes that lasts only six weeks, and then I shall snap back to boring blonde.

God has been good in that Ed has found temporary work for four weeks to help keep the wolf from the door and this Wednesday has an interview about a more permanent position, running a small tenant-improvement company for someone. Here's hoping!

My baby is so delightfully active now, especially when I get in the bath. As soon as the water starts running, the baby starts kicking. A doctor explained that water carries sound loudly, and this is why the splashing faucets agitate the baby. But it makes me sad to think what abortion does to these vibrant little babies. A doctor here in town advertises in the yellow pages for abortions up to twenty-four weeks. At twenty-five weeks my baby can obviously hear and react to outside sounds. He sleeps and wakes regularly, hiccups and may suck his thumb. Only a woman carrying a baby can relate to the humanity of the unborn child and the cruelty of abortion, which—

given without benefit of anesthesia—burns the baby's skin or tears him limb from limb. It's appalling. As someone remarked, "If the womb had windows, abortion would be illegal."

Speaking of the humanity of the baby, I recall nine years back, when I was carrying Luke in the third trimester, our alarm clock went off one morning, causing the baby literally to jump in fright. And once, when Hannah was inside me, I was drinking from a porcelain mug in the bathtub and accidentally knocked the side of the bath, causing a loud, underwater bang that made her jump. My whole stomach bounced with her shocked reaction!

Tuesday, February 22

I took the kids shopping at Wal-Mart and Toys "R" Us today, but my legs were giving out. I get a sharp pain like a burning fire behind my right knee, just as I did when I carried Hannah seven years ago. This, coupled with the pain in my groin when I walk a lot, makes me hopeless for long shopping ventures. Luke was looking for a basketball with me standing on one leg telling him, "Hurry up. I have to get out of here and sit down." I have tried to explain to the kids that pregnant women are often irritable, and they will have to be patient with me.

I bought some maternity trousers at Wal-Mart for thirteen dollars. This is so much cheaper than buying them at my designer maternity store. That is one benefit of being unemployed. It sets your priorities straight. No more browsing in pricey stores for me.

Week Twenty-Six

How is the baby doing?

The baby now weighs almost two pounds and measures about fourteen inches. He looks very much like a newborn infant and has the well-developed grip common to newborns. His eyelids are fused together, but in the next week or two they will open up, so that, for the rest of his sojourn in the womb, the baby will be able to open and shut his lids at will. If the baby were born prematurely now, he would have a good chance of surviving—he is "viable". However, he would have to spend several months in the hospital, with risks of infection and other complications. This week I could feel the baby kicking about two inches above my belly button, which shows the measurement of the uterus at this stage. In the next trimester my uterus will extend farther up to just below the breasts. In other words, it will occupy the whole abdomen.

The baby is, of course, surrounded by amniotic fluid, which he swallows and which acts as a buffer, protecting him from knocks. Doctors still do not know where the amniotic fluid comes from, but about one third of its volume is replaced every hour, so there is a daily fluid exchange of about six gallons at this stage of pregnancy. One theory is that the baby's lungs and kidneys produce the fluid, but this is unproved.

Monday, February 28

I had to take Luke into our new hospital facility for an X ray of the finger he broke playing football. Not wanting to hang around the X-ray area, Hannah and I left him to it and wandered upstairs to check out the nursery.

The maternity block is spanking new and beautiful. A nurse caught us having a sneaky look round an empty bedroom. I thought we'd get in trouble, but she was very nice and said she would look out for me in June. In the nursery were male twins born at 1 A.M.—very cute with striped ski caps on. Hannah and I drooled through the glass window and imagined that one day it would be our own precious baby lying in the nursery. How exciting!

The hospital offers a tour of the nursery, birthing room, delivery suite, etc., but it is an hour-and-a-half tour, and my legs get so sore now I don't want to be on my feet that long.

My doctor has suggested I do a Lamaze or Bradley childbirth class, but I don't think I'll bother. To be honest, I did a Lamaze course for my first baby and didn't find the breathing very helpful. I have always had a cynical mind, and I will bring down the wrath of the childbirth educators for saying this, but I think that childbirth is painful, and no form of fancy breathing is going to diminish the pain. Perhaps we can fool ourselves that by breathing slowly or puffing we can control the pain, but I didn't find it worked. As I said to Ed, "If someone is hammering a nail into your abdomen, no recipe for innovative breathing is going to make you feel good." Pain is pain. I told my doctor this, and he laughed. "You're too cynical", he said.

I laugh when I recall comedienne Joan Rivers' description of childbirth pain: "If you want to know what it feels like," she says, "you just take your bottom lip and pull it all the way over your head. That's what it feels like."

But, as Scripture tells us, the pain is soon forgotten when you hold the baby in your arms. In fact, with my second labor the pain was not too bad, and I managed well without any pain-relief drugs.

The Third Trimester

Week Twenty-Seven

Finally! I am into the third trimester. I feel like a racehorse on the home stretch. Weeks one though twelve are the first trimester; weeks thirteen through twenty-six are the second trimester; and twenty-seven to forty are the third. There is some leeway, however, because a normal birth (as opposed to a premature birth) is counted as anywhere from weeks thirty-eight through forty-two. Prior to thirty-eight weeks is "preterm", and after forty-two weeks is "post-term".

All my babies have been born three days before due date, so, since my due date is June 13, this would mean June 10, which is Ed's birthday and also (this year) the Feast of the Sacred Heart of Jesus. June 11 is the Feast of the Immaculate Heart of Mary. I would be thrilled to have a baby on either day.

Ten years ago, when I was pregnant with Luke (my first), Mom wrote me, quoting from Scripture, about how the grain of wheat must fall into the ground and die, or it remains but a single grain. But if it dies, it bears much fruit. She likened this to the mother during pregnancy.

Pregnancy is definitely a time of dying to self in order to bring forth new life. In the first trimester, there is the sickness and dizziness and sleeplessness; the second trimester is usually not too bad; and then the third trimester brings all the typical pains—swelling (edema), varicose veins, sometimes intermittent bleeding, backache, breast tenderness, shortness of breath, fatigue, hemorrhoids, heartburn, pelvic pains. Of course not all women experience all these symptoms (thank God!). Nevertheless, anyone who has carried a baby will relate to some of them. So I reflect on how apt Mom's Scripture selection was, and it helps me be more patient with my pregnancy. When I have died to myself, I shall truly bring forth new life. What a privilege!

Having said that—the old right thigh has truly blossomed with varicose veins right up near the groin, and they ache so badly they feel like fire and make it difficult to stand or walk any great distance. I have taken to strapping them with a piece of stretchy elastic to try to give additional support. I am so lucky to be an at-home mom, because when the pain gets bad I put my feet up on the couch for a while. I pity mothers who have to work. Imagine standing behind a shop counter for eight hours a day with throbbing leg veins! Working women are so courageous.

Monday, March 7

Last Saturday we felt like getting out of the house, so we went into San Francisco for the Chinese New Year's Parade. I ruined the expedition by limping and clinging to Ed for support. My thigh was throbbing so badly we gave up and hobbled back to the car. In spite of the pain, we had a good laugh. "It's like walking my ninety-year-old grandmother", Ed said. The sad thing is that my body feels healthy, and my mind is energetic—it's just that the skinny legs are not standing up to the weight of the baby. At this stage I have gained a total of sixteen pounds, which is average for this stage of pregnancy. I am trying not to stack on unwanted pounds, because it is more weight to carry around.

I had no complaints about my leg on Sunday after seeing my friend Donna, who is seven weeks ahead of me and in a wheelchair. Her poor hands are swollen to three times their size! She is forty-two, and this is her sixth baby. I turn forty-two next month and am grateful to be so active by comparison. She had toxemia (also called preeclampsia) in her fifth pregnancy (this is caused by high blood pressure and fluid retention), but her doctor assures her her swollen hands are just "normal" edema. She is such a good, patient, prayerful person. I pray she will have her baby early. I asked if I could take her two preschoolers to give her a break, but they are children who cry when separated from their mother, so she is reluctant to farm them out. This makes it difficult for her to get a good rest during the day.

I will be attending a baby shower for her next week. A friend offered to have one for me, but I said I would feel silly. I can't explain why, but Donna and I joke about being "geriatric mothers", and perhaps that is the reason . . .

Wednesday, March 9

We have been lucky. Having given away much of my baby equipment when I failed to get pregnant in the previous four years, I was wondering what to do. But a friend has offered us a crib, and today another friend brought over a playpen and a battery-operated swing. So I now have the three pieces I lacked. God is good. And people are generous.

Someone asked if we were "decorating a nursery" for the baby. I chuckled. That is something everyone does for the first baby, and it's fun. But by the fourth (or fifth, sixth, seventh), the baby just slots in wherever there is space. All the rooms are taken, so there is no separate nursery. Also, there is usually no money available to spend on decorations. This baby won't have a nursery at all but will probably just sleep with me. However, he will be smothered in love and attention, which may help compensate for the architectural deprivation of being "nursery-less".

WEEK TWENTY-EIGHT

Monday, March 14

My friend Donna was so swollen at the baby shower that a mutual friend drove her to the hospital, where they decided she did have toxemia after all. They held her there, tried to induce labor, and when that failed they took the baby by cesarean. Although he is six weeks premature, he weighed six pounds, and Donna is recovering nicely. Thank God her long ordeal is over!

I went to my obstetrician this week about my leg, which continually aches. He says he does not think it is a blood clot, but he told me not to wear the thigh bandage, as it was probably not helping. He told me to get a second opinion from my general practitioner. Last night my thigh veins were twitching in bed, so I shall take his advice and get a second opinion. While varicose veins are not a serious problem, a blood clot or thrombosis could be.

My weight has shot up this week, and I have now gained twenty pounds. It seems like a lot, but it is average for the twenty-eighth week.

We had bad and good financial news this week. You recall my visit to emergency in week twenty-one because of my fluttering heart? Well, the insurance company has refused to pick up the bill, which came to an astonishing $630. They say this is because I did not call my primary-care physician first to get his permission to go to emergency. I have written the medical review committee, stating that I was in contact with my obstetrician and that I think their decision unfair. Nevertheless, it is doubtful they will let us off.

The other bad news is that, although the insurance company originally told me they would pick up the

$350 fee for a labor coach, they now say they will not. So, if I want a coach to tell me when to go to the hospital, etc., I will have to pay that fee, too. This is turning into an expensive little baby. "You'd better be a great kid", I tell my stomach. "You're bankrupting us before you even arrive."

We finally had some good news about the job search. A small tenant-improvement company has offered Ed a position helping run the company. He will have to bring in jobs to bid and generally try to turn things around so it will make a profit. It is not exactly a "stable" job, considering the volatile state of construction right now, but if he makes a go of it, it will keep us in food . . . if not in mink coats. We were half way through a thirty-day novena to Saint Joseph (protector of the Holy Family) when he got the offer, so we must finish the novena as a thanksgiving prayer now.

Week Twenty-Nine

Monday, March 21

Bad luck again this week. The company that offered Ed the job has retracted it. The owner thinks he will close up shop after all, because the present climate is so unfavorable to construction. This is a blow, and poor Ed is back on the phones, job-hunting.

He was laughing at me last night because, when I am lying on the couch watching TV at night, I have taken to rolling off the couch and falling onto the floor on all fours like a dog. From that ungainly position, I then stand up. I find this easier than trying to sit up.

"Is this the lovely young thing I married?" he chuckles.

"Shall I strap a cannonball onto your stomach and see if you can do sit-ups?" I retort. It's hard to use your stomach muscles when they are compressed under all that weight. Plus, my stomach goes into a cone shape if I do, and I wonder what that does to the poor baby . . .

I saw my primary-care doctor this week, and he said the leg fibrillations are caused by the valves in the veins not being able to close properly because the veins have widened. He says it is not a catastrophe, and my veins will return to normal after the birth.

This week I also visited the midwife. Ed came with me. She said the baby is a perfect size for six and a half months but that my iron count has fallen drastically, so I have to go on iron pills. I hate these, as they make me constipated, so I am now drinking Metamucil fiber at night to counteract the effect of the pills. The joys of pregnancy!

The other pregnancy trauma I have now (which is a common one) is that if I cough or laugh really hard, I leak a little urine. This is because of the pressure of the baby on the bladder. I have experienced it in prior pregnancies, and the bladder always returns to its normal, efficient functioning after delivery. In the meantime, it is a good Lenten penance. I must stay away from people who make me laugh!

My girlfriend Sue came to pick up her little girl one evening and was shocked that I was limping and that I had to sit on a bar stool to prepare dinner. I was having a bad-leg day. If I can get ten hours in bed at night, my leg does better; but if I have only six or seven hours, my leg kills me from the time I get out of bed. But still . . . I keep rejoicing that I am in perfect health—no headaches, edema, bladder infections, heartburn, toxemia or other problems that many women suffer.

I keep complaining about aches and pains, so maybe it's worth reflecting on the subject of pain and suffering during pregnancy and labor. Are they a waste of time? The Church teaches that suffering has redemptive value, that in some mysterious way Christ, through his suffering and death, redeemed the world. The Church tells us to unite our sufferings to those of Christ on the Cross. I often tell my kids, "Don't waste your sufferings. Offer them up to save souls." Pregnant women do suffer, and it's important for us to make our suffering "useful" by giving it to God.

I heard of a priest who told a man in the hospital, "I'll pray for your healing."

"Oh, don't do that, Father", the man said. "My pain is all I have to offer him." How wonderful if we could all view our pain in this positive light.

Sister Faustina, the Polish nun recently beatified by

Pope John Paul II, wrote in her book *Divine Mercy in My Soul* (Stockbridge, Mass.: Marian Press, 1987): "Oh, if only the suffering soul knew how much God loves it, it would die of joy and of an excess of happiness! One day we shall know the value of suffering, but then we will no longer be able to suffer. The present moment is ours." I often read this when I am tempted to think negatively about my current problems.

I turned forty-two this week, and Luke is turning ten. I foolishly agreed to let him have a sleep-over pizza party for four friends, so I am sure we will be having all-night Nintendo games. Ah, well . . . I'll push Ed out of bed to shake a stick at them.

Luke's birthday is on the Feast of the Annunciation (March 25), and we made the effort to go to morning Mass as a family before school began. I felt so thankful to God for having given us Luke ten years ago. He is such a good little boy and has been a blessing to our family. There is no excitement quite like that first pregnancy, and no baby quite as spoiled as the first. But this pregnancy, coming after a six-year gap, is almost as exciting as a first, and now the other children are mature enough to share our excitement.

WEEK THIRTY

Monday, March 28

As I approach my eighth month, I feel tired (I got four hours sleep during Luke's slumber party, which didn't help!), something I didn't feel very much in the second trimester. Sometimes, by six at night, I feel I could collapse on the bed and die. I usually retire at 8 or 9 P.M. but then am up at 2 A.M. to relieve my bladder. Sometimes after this I lie awake worrying about whether Ed will find work, and then, when my alarm goes off at 7 A.M., I am exhausted. But last night I got ten hours uninterrupted sleep and woke feeling I could run a marathon. Could the Michelin tire man run a marathon?

Ed has two interviews this week, which is a miracle, since the San Francisco Bay area is so dead, but his résumé reads well, and we are grateful to get these interviews. He had phoned Seattle and Portland, but the companies there just laugh. "We have no work", they tell him. Boeing's latest closures and lay-offs in Seattle have left many engineers out of work. Anyway, we would be happier to find work here, as we have good friends in the area.

Someone asked if we were going to videotape the birth. I know the modern trend is to photograph or videotape every contraction, including the baby's head emerging from the vagina, but, as Ed says, "Blimey!

Who could you show them to?" And I agree. I don't think having a baby necessitates surrendering all modesty, and I don't want the whole world or even my children watching what is essentially a private function. Ed attends in the delivery room (some couples bring children in too, but we think this would be a horrific experience for children), but he just sits up by my head. "I like to stay clear of the boiler room", he tells the obstetrician. And he does not go in for the latest fad of having the dad cut the cord. "What are we paying these guys for?" he asks.

New Zealand men are different from American men—more macho, more embedded in the traditional male role, intolerant of feminism, not eager to trespass into the female domain. Having babies is woman's work to most "Downunder" men, and, probably because I hail from the same place, that is fine with me. I'd be uncomfortable with a feminist husband. Although I do wish he would give me an occasional back rub during labor. That wouldn't be too much to ask. . . .

Speaking of horrific photos, a girlfriend offered to give me her Bradley childbirth book when we were visiting them. The photos were gruesome. All the women were stark naked (why must one reveal one's breasts during childbirth, since they are not part of the action?), and the men—"partners" as they are called—were also semi-naked. The men, clad in rough-looking jeans, were kneeling or standing with their naked partners, usually the woman's legs spread wide open for the camera. I was amazed. "No, thanks", I told my girlfriend. "Naked butts spoil my appetite."

The level of vulgarity in some of these childbirth books is offputting. And yet in others the women are photographed looking beautiful, feminine, modest, and the mystery of delivery is preserved.

I would worry about bringing little children into delivery. Surely the sight of their mother in pain would put some little girls off having babies? There is trauma and suffering in labor that children should be spared.

I watched my dad deliver a baby when I was twenty years old and about to do a volunteer year in Western Samoa. Dad thought it would be good for me to learn about birth, because one of the nuns I would be assisting delivered babies in the village huts. At this mature age I found the experience fascinating. In fact, when the head emerged, I was reduced to tears of awe. It seemed like such a miracle, one life emerging from another. But I'm not sure at four or five years old I would have felt the same way.

Week Thirty-One

How is the baby doing?

The baby now weighs three and a half pounds and measures about eighteen inches. From twenty weeks to thirty weeks, the baby increased his weight five times. From thirty weeks to forty weeks, he will more than double his weight. His movements are so strong the mother feels her ribs are bruised with all the kicking. The baby now has eyebrows and eyelashes and longish hair, if he is the hairy type. His body has become plump and round, and his brain is well developed.

At some stage during the eighth month, many women experience a sudden lightening sensation as the baby drops down into the pelvis (I, personally, have never noticed it, but most of my friends say they have). At this point, the uterus sinks down about two inches, and the baby's head engages into the correct birth position. It is now only four and a half inches from being born, but what a battle lies ahead to move the baby that four and a half inches!

How is mom doing? I have got my pelvic pains back. As I mentioned before, this is caused by the pelvic joints becoming loose and lax so that the pelvic cavity will expand slightly and let the baby's head pass through at birth. This occurs more in older women and women who have had multiple births.

Wednesday, April 6

This morning I decided to go to the mall to buy a maternity belt to help support my abdomen. My obstetrician said this might help, although the midwife is against it, as she thinks the belts weaken the abdominal muscles. Anyway, I hate being inactive so will try the belt regardless.

I chuckled in the mall. As I was waddling along, each step causing me pain, a pregnant girl in her twenties strode past me at one hundred miles per hour, obviously feeling no pain. "She looks glorious", I thought. "She feels glorious. I hope she has quintuplets."

WEEK THIRTY-TWO

Tuesday, April 12

Ed is still unemployed. He had four interviews this week, but most companies are in no hurry to employ in this market. The only lively place for construction work is Los Angeles, and though we are loath to move there, it may come to that.

The 160-mg iron pills I had to take for anemia are still making me constipated, so I continue taking Metamucil every second day. This is harmless to the baby and helps the mom achieve some regularity. I am still taking my prenatal vitamins, about four a day. I usually take the iron at night when I get up to use the bathroom. If you take the iron too close to the vitamins, the vitamin E negates the iron. My energy level is good, although during the Easter break I took advantage of having the kids off school and slept till nine each morning. This week we are back to 7-A.M. starts.

I'm ashamed to admit I bought the *National Enquirer* this week because there was a front-cover picture of Vanna White, the "Wheel of Fortune" letter-turner, and I knew she was due to have her first baby a week ahead of me. Women often follow with interest other women whose babies are due at the same time. [Later on, I read she gave birth the same day I did.]

At seven months Vanna had gained about twenty-five pounds, which is about what I have now gained, but there the similarity ends. Vanna said she has had a very easy pregnancy, so she is obviously not waddling, as I am. She knows she is having a boy, but we have had no tests done and don't know what I am carrying.

She and husband George Santo Pietro are painting the baby's nursery blue and have racks of new baby clothes hanging in the baby's closet. Our baby has no nursery and only about five old nightgowns left over from the other children. I hope Vanna will not be placing her newborn in a separate nursery. Newborns should be right alongside the mother, preferably in her bed or in a crib alongside her bed so she can monitor him during the night. That way she can attach him to the breast the moment he cries. Babies love the closeness of the mother's body, which is why those snugglies that tie the baby onto the mom's body while she does housework are a great idea. Third-world women have known this for centuries and have always tied their babies to them with sarongs, lava lavas and other long strips of cloth.

Vanna says, "The crib and all the baby furniture are on order. Hopefully they'll be delivered by the end of April." Unfortunately, there won't be any Bloomingdale's trucks pulling into the Arnold driveway to deliver furniture. We have been given a baby swing and playpen, and a friend has an old crib in her attic that we have yet to pick up. With Luke I had a changing table too, but now we are cramped for space, so I shall skip the changing table and just change diapers on our bed.

Vanna says she and her husband talk to the baby and play music for him. "Every time we buy him a new toy or new piece of clothing, we describe it to him", she says. I think every mother talks to her unborn. I have told mine if he is a ten-pounder I shall smack his bottom when he emerges. And I say, "Hey, cut it out!" when the baby begins an aerobics program at midnight. Or I tell him, "Quit putting on weight. You're killing your old mother", as I use the bannister to drag myself upstairs at night. The children often put their little faces up to my stomach and tell the baby things: "I have a great doll house you can share when you come out." Or "We're having lasagna tonight. You'll love it." At Mass, during the kiss of peace, Laura always kisses my abdomen.

It's interesting reading about famous women preparing for motherhood. But, as with many babies born into larger families, what this baby lacks in the way of a Harrods-of-London nursery, the family will make up for in love and attention. As long as Ed can find work, I will be a full-time mother to him, and he has three siblings who will no doubt be fighting to have a turn at carrying him around. Babies born to ordinary families are just as cherished (maybe more so) than those born to the rich and famous.

WEEK THIRTY-THREE

Tuesday, April 19

During my visit to the doctor this week, he told me to try to slow my weight gain. I have gained twenty-six pounds, and doctors like you to keep to thirty pounds by delivery date, which doesn't leave me much more room for expansion.

This week I noticed some white discharge, but the doctor says this is normal and caused by the increased blood flow to the skin and muscles around the vagina. Another symptom that often accompanies this is called "Chadwick's sign", where the increased blood flow causes the vagina to turn a violet or blue color. From here until week thirty-six, I have a doctor's visit every two weeks and, after that, weekly visits until the birth.

I have started counting backward now—seven weeks left; six weeks left, etc. This is the exciting time.

Our friends kindly brought the crib over. It is a lovely white one, and they brought bedding to go with it, including a teddy-bear comforter. Spoiled baby!

We had bad luck on the job hunt this week. Ed got two offers—one from a small company he would have loved to work for and one from a large company that was an hour's commute away and he was not so enthusiastic about. He ended up losing both offers! The small company decided they need to wait a few months till construction picks up, and in the meantime he had asked the large company for twenty-four hours to make up his mind, and the boss got miffed with this and gave the job away! So Lady Luck deserted us. We have begun a nine-day rosary novena now to see if Our Lady can hurry things along.

This week I applied for the free lunch program at the school. The kids will be thrilled. Now they can have hamburgers, burritos and Kentucky Fried Chicken instead of my boring old peanut-butter sandwiches, so there are benefits to unemployment after all.

I remind myself that God is in control of the pregnancy—there is nothing I can do (or even know) about my baby's progress inside my womb. And God is in control of the unemployment too. When you have your college degree and your career, you feel you can control your destiny. Then you discover that everything is a gift of grace. And so we keep praying, "Jesus, I trust in Thee."

Week Thirty-Four

Monday, April 25

The last two nights when I have gotten up, the baby has gotten hiccups and kept up the rhythmic hics for ten minutes.

"Take a deep breath and hold onto it", I told the baby.

"Okay, Ma, but you cut out the glass of wine with dinner, and that will help me", the baby replied.

Then we both rolled over and went to sleep.

I was chuckling at a book I got out of the library, *Your Pregnancy Month by Month*, which was written back in 1977 by an obstetrician, Clark Gillespie. You can tell it is an older book because the doctor says things that modern doctors would never dare say, e.g.:

> What not to bring to the hospital—Do not bring bath towels, face towels or a bunch of relatives. Give any jewelry to your husband to take home. Remove heavy makeup and false eyelashes. If you wear contact lenses, leave them at home. Spit out your gum!

I laughed about the false eyelashes, which are not in vogue at all today, although they were in the seventies. And that the doctor *dared* to say not to bring relatives.

One thing that used to rile my dad when he was a practicing obstetrician was patients bringing all their relatives into the delivery room. Or their boyfriend and ex-boyfriend and a couple of giggling girlfriends. It got on my dad's nerves, because he felt as if he had a travelling circus breathing down his neck when he was trying to concentrate on delivering the baby. It probably bothers other obstetricians, too, to have hordes of people come in to watch a delivery, but today most would be too intimidated to object. It has become the patient's right to bring in whomever she wants.

Wednesday, April 27

Oh dear. I went to the midwife today for my thirty-four-week check-up, and she told me the baby is breech. Just my luck. But she says not to worry, as it still has time to turn to the head-down position, and, if it doesn't, the obstetrician will try turning it through external version. She suggested I go home and scrub the kitchen floor, as this sometimes causes a baby to perform a flip. She said the baby is "long", but she doesn't know if it will be another nine-pounder like my last one. The obstetrician will check the position again at my thirty-six-week visit.

WEEK THIRTY-FIVE

Tuesday, May 3

My weight has stabilized and is not increasing at such a fast rate, thank God. I am five foot seven inches and started the pregnancy at 145 pounds. I now weigh 170 pounds, so it is a twenty-five-pound weight gain, and I expect it will be thirty by the time I deliver, but they say that the baby doesn't grow much after week thirty-seven, and your weight tends to stabilize there.

My pelvic pains and the pains from the varicose veins in my groin and thigh area are much less than they were two months back, so I am lucky there, too. I'm actually doing better as I get larger. Now if only Ed could find work. . . . He is getting depressed with the lack of action, but underneath it all we both trust that God will find us something in his own time.

I heard a sad story this week about a good Christian couple having their third baby in a home birth. Home births have been very "in" during the last ten years as a kind of reaction against the overtreatment and overly restrictive atmosphere of the hospital. Also because of the high cost of hospital deliveries. Plus, many young couples are looking for a more holistic, natural life-style, and home birthing fits that philosophy.

Nevertheless, my father has always argued that home births put the baby's life at risk. Every birth is a potential emergency, and the only safe way of treating an emergency is in a hospital, Dad used to say. I don't find it hard to accept this, because there is so much that can go wrong during a birth that might necessitate an emergency cesarean. In the home-birth situation, it can take half an hour to get to the hospital and another half hour to fetch the doctor in and get set up for a cesarean operation. That is a good sixty minutes where the baby is without treatment.

This is exactly what happened to this couple in Washington State. They had had two previous successful home births with a midwife in attendance, but with this third baby, the baby got stuck in the birth canal, and the midwife was unable to deliver her. . . . By the time they did get to the hospital, the baby was brain dead. She was kept on life support for two days and then taken off it. What a tragedy, and for such a good couple, too!

Some of my friends swear by home births and will not accept that this is a potential risk for the baby. While the mother faces certain risks during delivery, the baby faces ten times as many risks. What can go wrong? Shoulder disproportion is not an uncommon delivery event. The head delivers, but the shoulders are trapped and require expert management to deliver with safety to both mother and child. This allows little time leeway. This may have been what happened in the case mentioned above.

Or sometimes there is a prolapsed cord, which can kill the baby within minutes unless aggressive treatment is used. Occasionally, a mother will hemorrhage badly after delivery, a situation that requires immediate hospital treatment. Or the baby might fail to start breathing and need to be put on a machine that is available only at the hospital.

Most obstetricians will not preside over a home birth because they are aware of the disasters that can occur. Statistics, too, show that it is safer to have a hospital birth. For example, in 1940, when 56 percent of deliveries occurred in hospitals, the infant mortality was forty-seven per thousand, and the maternal death rate 376 per hundred thousand. By 1980, 99 percent of deliveries were in hospitals, and the infant mortality rate had dropped to 12.4 per thousand and the maternal mortality rate to 6.9 per hundred thousand.

Women who have had one or two easy deliveries in the past think that they are "safe" candidates for home births, but figures from the National Center on Health Statistics show that 20 percent of women with no underlying medical conditions and no previous problems in pregnancy develop some problem during labor.

What a home birth mother *does* avoid is being a victim of this country's high cesarean rate. Nevertheless, as one mother said to me, "I would rather that I have to undergo an unnecessary cesarean section than that my baby die because I was unwilling to give birth in a hospital."

And you can lower your cesarean rate by shopping around for a doctor with a lower rate. Unfortunately, in my own experience, it is the older doctors (i.e., those over sixty) who usually have the lower surgical rates. As these doctors retire, we are left with fewer to choose from. The younger doctors seem to be trained to use cesarean section as the solution to simple obstetrical problems that their older peers would easily handle in a nonsurgical manner, e.g., by turning a breech manually or using forceps.

Week Thirty-Six

Tuesday, May 10

This week we are getting a third seat added to our Toyota Land Cruiser to accommodate our growing family. There is a company in Stockton, California, called Seats for Little People, and for four hundred dollars they are putting in the extra seat. They try to match the existing upholstery.

I was thinking this week about "bonding" because I told my obstetrician that I would like to nurse the baby immediately after birth. He said this was a good idea because it would help me to "bond" with the baby. Remember the bonding syndrome that was so much in vogue ten years ago? The parenting magazines were full of it. Mothers were told how important it was to "bond" with their newborns.

Cynic that I am, I was always sceptical about whether a psychological state called "bonding" existed. I considered the bonding activity just another example of psychobabble. After all, our mothers never heard of it, and many of us are very attached to our mothers.

Yuppies took their bonding seriously, but then a lot

of yuppie babies ended up in day care. A woman who worked in a local day-care center in our town told us that two female lawyers were dropping their six-week-old babies off at day care at 7 A.M., driving into their San Francisco offices and picking the babies up again at 7 P.M. Even the day-care workers thought this was heartless, because the newborns cried a lot during the day. But did the women lawyers believe they had "bonded" with their babies? I'm sure they did. They probably thought they gave their babies "quality time" rather than "quantity time".

Bonding is one of those "in" terms that doesn't appeal to me. I think the best mothers love their children in the sense that they are available to them, generous with their time and attention, physically affectionate, ready to sacrifice of themselves and their careers and material possessions, patient and always ready to comfort a child. I think your religion plays an important part in mothering, too. A Christian mother knows that she is the heart of the family and that she must lay down her life in one form or another for the sake of her children. Being a good mother is, to me, a spiritual, not a psychological, concept. After all, who is to say that a woman with no religious standards won't one day desert all her expertly bonded children and run off with the local plumber?

Ed drove up to Portland and Seattle this week looking for work there, as the San Francisco Bay area is still pretty dead. The day he left, I cried off and on all day, but I guess this is partly the pregnancy hormones. Pregnant women are definitely emotional. How lucky one is to have a husband's support during pregnancy and child-rearing, and how brave are all those single mothers who have to do it alone, especially when they are bombarded with offers of abortion as a way out.

I now have only four weeks to go. I am up twice a night to use the bathroom. My bladder has the capacity of the fuel tank on a toy truck—almost zero. Also, I perspire during the night, probably because my body has such a high metabolic rate now. Ed is shivering under the blankets, and I'm perspiring.

I spoke with a potential labor coach this week. We shall get together in two weeks to discuss the upcoming labor, in which she will help me through contractions.

I had some good news this week. *Readers Digest* will pick up a column I wrote and pay me nine hundred dollars for it! I am thrilled not only for the exposure in their publication (which, with one hundred million readers, is the world's most widely read magazine) but because this will help pay the mounting bills.

At this point of the pregnancy I am thinking about how nice it will be to fit into "normal" clothes again and to be slim. It usually takes me only a couple of months to get all the weight off, because breast-feeding strips all the calories out of me—it's the best weight-loss device in the world! I can never eat enough to cover the extra six hundred calories a day needed to breast-feed, and so it comes off me as fat.

My weight gain has slowed these past three weeks, and my total gain is now about twenty-seven pounds. Still, I was struggling in from the car yesterday, lugging three ten-pound packets of flour for our bread-making machine, and I thought: thirty pounds, what a huge weight to carry, and I am carrying it now as a result of the pregnancy.

Some girlfriends are throwing a shower for me after the baby arrives. I feel a bit silly, this being my fourth, but they insisted, and so I accepted. I think the women enjoy getting together. Certainly we won't say No to any offers of help in the face of our continued unemployment.

Friday, May 13

Today I visited the obstetrician, and he said he is positive the baby is no longer breech, so that is a relief. At this thirty-six week visit, it is usual for the doctors to do an internal check to see if there is any effacement or dilatation of the cervix. There was none. He said everything seemed fine. I asked him if he believed the story the midwife told me, that if I went home and scrubbed the floor the baby would probably right his breech position. He laughed and said, "That's pure voodoo." My dad says the same thing. Many women swear that certain exercises by the mother will cause a baby to turn, but my dad told me years back that there is nothing a woman can do externally to turn the baby around. "It's an old wives' tale", he said.

My children continue to delight me. When a neighbor was unpacking a new piece of furniture, the kids spied the five-foot-long carton it came in and asked for it. They dragged it home, and it became a house, a ship, a stretch limo. At night the girls dragged it up to their bedroom, Hannah dumped all her bedding into it, and she has been sleeping inside the box for two weeks.

At night Ed and I tell her, "Quiet down and go get in your box!" Their bedroom looks like a Bangladesh shanty town. I told Hannah, "You must get rid of the box and start sleeping in bed again, or I'll put stamps on your box during the night and mail you off to India." She reluctantly returned to the civilized world, and the box is out in the back yard.

Week Thirty-Seven

How is the baby doing?

The baby now weighs six and a half pounds and measures about twenty inches. He won't change much now except to grow and gain a little more weight before the day of the big push. Scalp hair is growing well, and the fingernails and toenails are probably ready for their first clipping. The baby's body will be covered with the waxy white vernix caseosa that protects it from the amniotic fluid. The last important thing the baby had to undergo was maturation of the lungs and respiratory system. This is always a concern with premature infants, that their lungs will be underdeveloped, but by this stage the lungs should be in good shape. The placenta reaches maximum efficiency at thirty-seven weeks and then gradually begins to deteriorate over the next few weeks.

I know there is nothing wrong with this baby's hearing, because I was in the bath last night and the baby became very agitated when the faucets were running. I talked soothingly to him to try to calm him down. As soon as I turned the faucets off, the baby immediately stopped moving.

I was tired and achy in the groin Monday because I was restless during the night and only got about five hours sleep. I hope I'm not this tired when I go into labor.

Tuesday, May 17

No job offers have come out of Portland or Seattle. Today Ed is interviewing in Reno, Nevada. It is stressful for him, but he is a good hustler, and I really admire him for not giving up the job search in these difficult conditions. If he finds work out of state, I might have to have the baby alone, but that would not worry me unduly. The main thing is for him to get settled into a job so he can support us all.

I have my own little breech test now, which I find reassuring (although doctors may not find it scientific!). Often at night, if I get up, the baby seems to awaken from my moving around and (I suspect) have a gulp of the amniotic fluid. Then, when I get back in bed, I can feel the baby hiccuping. The rhythmic hiccing comes from my lower abdomen, which I interpret to mean the baby's chest and throat area are down there. If the hiccing were coming from above my belly button, I would presume the baby was head up and therefore in the wrong position. While the observation interests me, it is also frustrating to have to suffer the baby's midnight hiccups.

This week's doctor's visit was uneventful. Baby still head down. At one point the doctor grabbed the baby's foot and said, "Here, hold this. It's the foot."

"How gross", I laughed. There is something extra-terrestrial about feeling someone else's body parts inside one's body.

My weight is now 176 pounds, so I have gained thirty-one pounds, which is okay with the doctor but not with me. My poor skinny legs are giving out!

WEEK THIRTY-EIGHT

Only three more weeks to go. I can't believe it. This is the time when moms are ready to give up and pack the whole thing in. These last few weeks are the staggering weeks, when the only thing worse than the thought of having to go through labor is the thought of having to go on carrying this sack of flour in your midriff. Nights now are broken with two or three toilet visits, as the bladder gives up under the weight of the pressure. I sometimes go to the bathroom and then ten minutes later rush back again, but it is more the baby's head than the pressure of urine that gives one that desperate feeling.

Tuesday, May 24

This morning, after dropping the kids at school at 9 A.M., I came home and lay down on the bed and didn't awaken till noon. I felt great the rest of the day. In my last week I'll try to nap often in preparation for the big push.

Ed got work this week, although it is not very satisfying. The man who initially offered a job and withdrew it twenty-four hours before he began called and reoffered the position. He will take Ed on for three months to see if he can turn the small construction company around so it shows a profit. If it does, Ed could eventually take over the company, but it is a complex, risky situation. Then last night we had a call from one of the companies in Portland that he had visited, and they want to fly him up for a second interview, so he will fly up on June 5 to talk with them. Poor Ed isn't keen on the trip, but we decided it is better to talk to all comers in case something better comes up. Portland has cheaper houses but lots of rain.

And how would I manage a move and house hunting with the baby? It doesn't pay to think about it. One day at a time is the rule right now.

I met with the girl who will be my labor coach this week. She seems pleasant. Her charge is a bit high—$375—but she kindly said I can pay what I think is fair, seeing as we have been unemployed. She told me the hospital has private Jacuzzi tubs in each room, and the women often labor in them. You can direct a Jacuzzi jet onto painful back-labor areas. My first three babies were all posterior, which causes back labor. Maybe this one is, too. Anyway, it appeals to me, as I love baths. She said to call her when I know I am in labor and she will be there in a half hour. She will help direct me in breathing, give back rubs, advise me on position changes, etc. I found back rubs helpful with my second baby.

I have been having constant Braxton Hicks contractions. One night this week I got my p.v.c.s (premature ventricular contractions) back, which was disappointing. I was tired and stressed and having contractions, and my heart started the old pounding/jumping routine. The doctor said if this happens during labor to come to the hospital earlier than I had intended, and they may be able to give me something to quiet my heart. I would definitely find it distracting having p.v.c.s throughout labor. But that is in God's hands. We trusted in him, and he found work for Ed, and now we place the safe delivery of our baby into his loving hands.

Week Thirty-Nine

Monday, May 30—Memorial Day

Fourteen more days till due date, and hopefully it will come earlier, as my other three did. No wonder women hate the last two weeks—you feel so heavy, tired and uncomfortable.

I took the girls to the mall this morning to buy Ed a shirt for his birthday (June 10). My legs ached so badly I had to keep sitting down. I have gained one more pound: total weight now up from 145 to 177 and my poor legs feel like they are going to snap. We grabbed a shirt and then went upstairs, where I intended buying an engagement present for a young friend, but I could feel a grouch attack coming on. I felt like snapping at the girls and had to sit down on a gorgeous $1,500 display couch. "Will they make me buy it if my water breaks?" I wondered. I quickly perused the china department and then said, "Let's hit the car while I can still walk."

It is best to stay close to the house and just rest up at this stage. I have my overnight bag packed with nightie and baby clothes and a toilet bag with toothbrush and some makeup. I can't think what else I might need.

I'm wondering if the baby has "dropped", because I can never tell, except that I am not so puffed, but I still have terrible gas and can eat only small meals, after which I burp a lot. Some women get heartburn, which I have never experienced, but the constant burping is unpleasant. Fortunately, we can't afford to go to restaurants, or I'd have people moving their tables away from me!

Tuesday, May 31

My visits to the doctor are weekly now. The doctor told me he will be at a conference in San Francisco on the tenth, eleventh and twelfth—just the days I am expecting the baby to appear. It is an hour's drive away, and he says he will try to get back for the birth. I hope so, or the baby will be delivered by a stranger.

It pays to have prolife friends. My friend Bev, who helps at the crisis pregnancy center, gave me three bags full of gorgeous baby clothes—they are all girl's clothes. Does this mean I am having a girl? The Lord provides. I started out with nothing for this baby, having given everything away, and now the baby has better clothes and a nicer crib than the other three had—all contributed by friends. People are so sweet, especially when they know you are unemployed.

My girlfriend Donna was sitting in front of us at Sunday Mass with her baby, so we got to hold him after Mass. Laura and Hannah were smitten. I have two eager babysitters. It is always hard to believe a baby will actually emerge. Having lived with this growing lump for nine months, it still seems a miracle that a real, unique child exists within me. I don't know if other women feel this way, but I often find it hard to believe there is a baby there. Intellectually I know there is, but emotionally I can't quite grasp it—not until the doctor hands me the baby, and I see him with my own eyes. . . . The creation of a life is such a mysterious thing. Is this why Doubting Thomas wanted to touch Christ's wounds? Where does life come from? How does it get here? I think I would have wanted to touch the Lord's wounds, too . . .

Week Forty

The final week . . . the final lap . . . the last leg. And none too soon. This is when mother is literally dragging herself around the house and the supermarket, the weight of her little Siamese twin getting more oppressive each day. Or perhaps it's just my age. Perhaps women in their twenties are still light on their feet . . .

Saturday, June 4

Last night I fell asleep at 9 P.M., then got up to use the bathroom at 11 P.M., then again at 3:45 A.M., and the dog woke me with its barking at 5:00 A.M. Ugh.

It's important for first-time moms to realize that, as the due date nears, it is vital to get a lot of sleep in preparation for delivery. With my first baby, I was up at 5 A.M. to cook Ed's breakfast, and it was a stupid thing to do, as I had a forty-hour labor that began that same day, and I was exhausted. So tell your husband to look after his own breakfast as the time nears. You need all the sleep you can get.

A friend who was going to be induced for her first baby went to the ballet the night before and sat around chatting excitedly with her husband till the wee small hours. She failed to get any sleep the night before being induced, ran out of energy and had a cesarean. The mother should be like an athlete in training this week, and one of the most important things is early nights. They don't call it "labor" for nothing.

Sunday, June 5

We all went to the library today. I wanted to stock up on books for the kids to keep them occupied when junior arrives. Sheila Kitzinger has put out a new book on *Birth at Home*, and I was alternatively appalled and amused by the graphic photos of women delivering at home. One is of a hugely fat woman (around 250 lbs.) with breasts to sink the Titanic, giving birth in a bath in her home. She is wallowing in the tub like a trapped whale—definitely not a product of the Ford Modeling Agency! The photos made me grin. The fat woman in the bath (who is probably a very nice person) delivered a baby called Sam. What will Sam think when presented in future years with this graphic memorial of his birth? Will he proudly pass it around his baseball team or incinerate it?

Wednesday, June 8

Good news at this morning's doctor's visit. I am two centimeters dilated, and most labors start with the woman between one and three centimeters dilated, so within the next few days we might see some action. All of those Braxton Hicks, softening-up contractions have finally achieved something.

The doctor was teasing me because he has a conference in San Francisco and doesn't want to be called back for the birth. "You probably have another six weeks to go", he said. Then he laughed and admitted the cervix had softened and I might be close to delivering.

Thursday, June 9

What a disappointing day! My contractions grew stronger last night. I had a show of blood at 11 P.M., then the mucus plug dropped out when I went to the bathroom at 4 A.M., and I thought that labor was really picking up. But it didn't. In the morning it dropped off. By afternoon I was getting around three or four good painful contractions an hour, but they were not getting stronger or closer together. How disappointing. I thought with my fourth baby I would start labor and have a nice accelerated pace, but I am having an on-again, off-again time. I got about five hours broken sleep last night and am feeling tired today—not a good way to face labor when it gets under way. The only good part is that tomorrow is Ed's birthday and the Feast of the Sacred Heart, so it would be a prestigious day to give birth.

Friday, June 10

Awakened at 1 A.M. by stronger contractions. At 2:30 A.M. I woke Ed, and we went downstairs to have a cup of tea. It was nice sitting in the darkened living room, wondering if the baby was actually coming. Ed is eager for it to be born on his birthday. I snuggled into Ed's arms and laid my head on his chest. It was a comforting time—the calm before the storm.

We went back to bed, and I dozed for a while. By 4:30 A.M. my contractions were coming one after another and getting stronger, so I called my coach. She arrived by 5:30 A.M., but then a strange thing happened. (My midwife later told me she thought it was due to "performance stress"—in other words, you've awakened the coach, this had better be the real thing!) When she arrived, my contractions stopped. Just like that. Nothing. Zero. Zilch. I had one strong contraction during the half hour she was here. She decided I was too cheerful to be dilated at all, so she left at 6:00 A.M., saying she would call me around 11 A.M. to see if they had picked up. Ed wondered if he should go to work, but I asked him to wait an hour.

Just as well! I went upstairs to bed, feeling disappointed, but as soon as I fell into the bed, the contractions began again, sharply and one on top of the other. By 6:30 A.M., the pain was becoming unbearable. I staggered into the bathroom, where I stood leaning on the countertop and groaning. This was the real thing, and I felt the baby might be close to being born.

I will never understand how I so successfully shut down my labor when the coach arrived. My father claims women have no control over their uterine contractions, but this experience convinced me we do. I think I wasn't altogether comfortable with this coach. I didn't have the strong bond I had had with the first coach, the one I had when delivering Laura. In some way I found her presence off-putting. And, as the midwife said, I felt under a lot of stress to perform, not only because Ed wanted the baby born on his birthday but because I had gotten the coach out of bed at an ungodly hour. Anyway, it was a blessing in disguise, because as it turned out the coach would have been superfluous because of the constant presence of the midwife. (Staying throughout labor and delivery is a mark of the midwife, unlike the obstetrician, who just comes in occasionally to check progress.) Plus it saved me the $375 fee. Well . . . $295, because I later mailed the coach eighty dollars to thank her for her two visits to my house. She wrote back an appreciative note.

Anyway, back to the labor . . .

I called out to Ed to phone our friends who would

come and mind the still-sleeping children. Then I gave myself a Fleets enema. My doctor doesn't believe in enemas, but the thought of pushing out a bowel movement, as often happens when women are pushing the baby out, did not appeal to me. Also, I had read that an empty bowel makes the passage of the baby easier. And I'm all for clearing the decks for an easy passage! The enema worked immediately, and I was relieved that I would be going to the hospital with an empty bowel.

By this time Luke and Laura were up and timidly watching me from the bathroom door as I continued holding on to the countertop and groaning loudly.

"Are you okay, Mom?" Laura asked nervously.

"I'm fine, darling. This is just normal for having a baby."

Ten minutes had passed since I had first staggered to the bathroom. Ed called the midwife. (Sure enough, the obstetrician was away at the conference.) The midwife claims you can tell how dilated a woman is by the sound of her voice. The previous evening she said I didn't sound as if I was in hard labor.

"How are you doing, Mary?" she asked.

My voice came out a desperate whine. "I think I'm about to have it", I groaned.

This time there was no mistaking my progress.

"Get to the hospital quickly", she said. "I'll see you there."

I descended the stairs, hanging onto Ed for support. At times like this I appreciate my big bear of a husband. Ed had the Land Cruiser with engine running, and I climbed painfully inside as soon as Larry and Susan pulled up in their pickup truck. Larry squeezed my hand.

"Good luck, darling", Susan said. "We'll feed the kids and get them off to school. They'll be fine." I was grateful for their support.

The six-minute ride to the hospital was painful, and I raised my hips off the seat every time Ed stopped for a light or turned a corner. For some reason that seemed to ease the pain. "I think I'm in transition [I wasn't]. I think I'm going to have it in the car", I told Ed. He stepped on the gas.

At the hospital I was taken by wheelchair up to a cheerfully decorated delivery room, where my midwife, who had just arrived, said I was six centimeters dilated. This was great news!

"If you don't take any drugs, you'll be holding your baby in about ninety minutes", she told me.

Call me a coward, call me gutless, but with contractions coming now in violent waves, one on top of the other, ninety minutes sounded like ninety hours. I told her an epidural sounded very good. If I'd been giving birth where there were no drugs, I'd have gotten through it, but where relief is available, it is often too tempting to pass up. So they gave me a "light narcotic" (doesn't that sound good?) epidural that wore off gradually. Then they added a pitocin drip, because the epidural slows the labor contractions and pitocin speeds them up again. I had reached the hospital at 7:30 A.M. By 11 A.M. the epidural was wearing off, so I could feel my contractions again.

At 10 A.M. (fortunately before the epidural wore off), I went through transition, and it was like nothing I had experienced before. My body started shaking like the body of a rag doll in the hands of an angry child. My hands shook violently, as did my arms, chest and abdomen, my entire body. Although I felt no pain, I thought I must be dying. I suspected something had gone wrong with the epidural. I had visions of an air bubble getting into my system, and I felt I was about to explode. Ed looked horrified.

"What's wrong with me?" I asked the nurse.

"You've hit transition. It's normal for some women to shake a lot while going through it", she said, assuring me my vital signs were all right.

"Stop shaking", Ed said.

"I can't. I've lost control of my body."

After about twenty minutes, the shaking subsided, to my relief. Apparently, shaking really is a normal part of transition (related to the release of adrenalin in your body) for some women, but I had never experienced it.

The midwife kept checking my dilation. At one point she saw the baby's head and told me it was bald. Then she checked fifteen minutes later and said it was a hairy baby. She had made a mistake. At 11 A.M., only the rim of the cervix remained, and she started helping me by massaging the cervix outward with her fingers.

At 11:15 she told me to push, which I did, although it was hard, as I felt no urge to push. By 11:25 I did feel the urge, which helped me.

The midwife told me to hold onto my knees to bring my body forward as I pushed, but I was too weak to do it. She wanted my legs spread farther apart, but I couldn't hold them open so Ed held one knee open and a nurse forced the other knee open as I pushed. I found the pushing painful. With previous births I had found it a relief and not painful at all. Perhaps with advanced age the whole birth process is more difficult. I pushed hard for forty-five minutes. The midwife was wonderful.

"You're doing great", she kept saying. "You're a wonderful pusher."

I knew I was a lousy pusher, but I appreciated her encouragement. She was like a guardian angel through the whole ordeal. I couldn't have hoped for a lovelier person as a coach.

At this point the head nurse, whom I had found less sympathetic than the other staff, did something totally zany. She stood between my open legs and asked me, "Do you want champagne or apple cider in your Congratulations Basket?" (She was referring to a complimentary basket the hospital gives women after the birth—a little public-relations gesture.)

I couldn't believe she was asking me something so trivial when I was desperately trying to give birth. Laboring women often become rude and obnoxious. I opened my mouth to say, "Drop dead." Instead, I grunted, "Speak to her, Ed." Ed said, "Champagne." As she wandered off again, I thought, "I hope you get run over by a train, and, in your death throes, a passerby asks you, 'Do you want a marble headstone or a brass plaque?' "

The obstetrician came in at 11:50 A.M. He was my doctor's locum, and I had never met him, but at this point I couldn't have cared less. Suddenly I could feel the baby's head like a huge melon in my vagina. It felt bizarre, and I wanted it out of there. But fast.

(I should mention at this point that pushing can be a noisy business. I don't consider myself all that noisy, and I don't scream during labor, but if a woman wants to shout and puff loudly, she should be able to. When I was laboring with Laura, I had a nurse tell me to "Quiet down." I think this is callous. It didn't happen this time.)

"One more push and I'll have the head", the doctor said. I pushed again. The head and shoulders were born.

"The baby's here", Ed cried out, a bit prematurely. I pushed with all my might, and the whole body shot out into the doctor's hands.

It was one minute before noon on Ed's birthday and the Feast of the Sacred Heart, June 10.

Then I amazed myself by giving a howl of victory that filled the delivery room. It was a shout of release, of accomplishment, of triumph. It was an animal reaction. I hadn't planned it. It was immediate and involuntary, and as I shouted I wondered, "Is that me?" The midwife assured me later that many women give a similar shout as the baby delivers. But it was such a strange, spontaneous, dramatic outburst. I'll never forget it.

"It's a girl", the doctor and Ed said in unison.

After declining the doctor's offer for him to cut the cord ("I'm not a midwife", Ed said ungraciously), Ed took her from the doctor and dropped her, all slippery-slimy and bloody onto my stomach.

Mary Elizabeth Arnold did what all babies do on this momentous occasion. She took a breath and yelled with rage. I kissed her slimy face and held her cheek against my cheek. She felt like a little, wet frog—looked like one, too. I tried attaching her to my bosom, but she was too angry, so I handed her, still yelling, to the nurse for clean-up.

For some reason I didn't burst into joyful tears, as I had when the doctor had dropped Hannah onto my belly seven years before. Perhaps her yells distracted me or reminded me that I would be up every night for the next few months quelling those howls. I was thrilled and excited to see her and finally hold her after all those months of carrying her invisibly, but I wasn't bowled over by a tidal wave of mother love. Every birth is different, and every reaction is different. Needless to say, I was thrilled to have her, my much-wanted and much-loved baby, and to see that she was normal.

In spite of the dire predictions, she was not Down's syndrome, and she was not handicapped in any way.

She was a perfect, gingery-haired, blue-eyed, ferocious little girl.

Five minutes later, with one easy push, the placenta delivered. The doctor had not performed an episiotomy, and I had a "first-degree" tear to the vagina, so while Mary Liz (yes, we'd opted for Mary, after the Mother of God) was performing her Apgar tests (she passed with flying colors), I watched in repugnance as the doctor injected some pain reliever and stitched me up with a huge fishhook-shaped needle.

"I presume the stitches will dissolve", I said, hopefully.

He assured me they would and that a first-degree tear was not a bad one.

At this point the nurse returned with our now non-slimy offspring. We noted that she had lots of gingery hair and was definitely an Arnold, resembling both Luke and Hannah. She weighed eight pounds, four ounces, and was nineteen inches long—a beautiful baby, the pediatric nurse assured us, although we weren't convinced. I mean . . . she was exquisite in our eyes but, objectively speaking, was definitely plain. (Laura, with her huge, wide-open eyes, had been my most beautiful newborn.)

I tried suckling her again, but she was still too distracted, and it wasn't until four hours later in the hospital bed that I finally got Mary Liz to take my breast. She proved a fiercely capable nurser, shouting in temper as I changed her from one breast to the other. I was beginning to fall seriously in love with her. One forgets how lovely babies are, with their goofy, cross-eyed looks and the way they form a little "o" with their mouths.

Ed and the children were in the room with me for this first nursing, and it was a poignant moment. Ed had gone to school and picked them up. When they were all belted up in the car, he told them, "You have a . . . [leaving them in torment for ten seconds] *sister*!"

Luke was too excited to be disappointed that he didn't have the brother he'd longed for. When they saw her in the nursery crib in a funny little striped ski cap, there was no question she was what they wanted. "We'll get you a boy next time", I told him. Ed looked at me in horror. "After a few months, of course", I added.

That first nursing with the six of us all together as a family is locked in my memory as the high point of the birth. The children watched in reverent awe as the newest Arnold labored at the breast, one tiny hand resting on my bosom, her little, ginger head cradled in my arms, topped by the ridiculous ski cap that made the others laugh. We marveled at her loud sucking, and I praised God in my heart for this wondrous creation.

Conclusion

The end of this book is in sight, but concluding it now, four months after the birth, I might add several observations:

I did not get the p.v.c.s during labor. My heart performed perfectly. My legs, which had been so painful during pregnancy, returned immediately to their prepregnancy state, and I have no pain at all now. Even the varicose veins by my groin have disappeared.

Mary Liz proved to be a colicky baby, and, since we'd never had a baby with colic, it was a hair-raising experience. During weeks three and four of her life, she was out of control, crying nonstop for hours on end. We forced her to take a pacifier, and it was the only thing that ever quieted her. We tried all the tricks in the book: driving around the block at midnight, running the vacuum cleaner, using nonlactose soy milk, putting her on top of the washing machine, etc., etc. But nothing worked. Colic is wretched. It is apparently related to an immature digestive (and/or nervous) system, and it produces miserable babies. But friends and pediatricians assured us it would disappear overnight at the three-month stage. It did. Two weeks before she turned three months, she quieted down and began to enjoy life. So did we. At last. So, if you have a colicky baby, don't jump off a cliff. Sit on your husband's knee, sip a gin and have a good cry, but don't despair. At three months Mary Liz became a gorgeous, smiling, alert little angel who has brought us nothing but joy ever since.

We had her baptized on day nine by our good friend, Father Terry Tompkins. With the other babies, we had waited five weeks, until I was strong enough to host a christening party, but with this one we decided to skip the party, just invite the godparents and get the job done. It was a relief to know she was now in a state of perfect grace.

I have come to realize it's okay not to breast-feed fully. I found that at age forty-two total breast-feeding was leaving me weak and frail. I felt so drained that after three months I started supplementing, and immediately my energy returned. I felt guilty for not offering 100 percent breast milk, but sometimes mom needs to think of herself, too. Total breast-feeding suited me fine in my thirties, but at forty-two I found it was just too much for me. Heck, some women are grandmothers at forty-two—I shouldn't feel guilty. Now, at four months, she is happily on formula and only breast-fed once or twice a day. It was a compromise, but it gave me back my strength.

The baby brought us a blessing. A month after she was born, Ed switched jobs. He now works as the construction manager for a large amusement park that spends about ten million dollars a year building new rides and refurbishing old ones. I have never seen him so happy with a job. It's like nothing he has ever done before. It's more fun than building office buildings.

Plus, we get free season passes, so I'm putting Mary Liz on a fifty-foot roller coaster to repay her for my labor pains. Just kidding, folks.

I had forgotten the joy that a baby sprinkles like fairy dust wherever she goes. I cannot go to Mass or the supermarket or the library without perfect strangers coming up to ogle the baby. If I go to the market without the baby, no one smiles at me or notices me. With the baby, we are instant celebrities. We attract an entourage. The other day a handsome young man in a suit and tie came over to the shopping cart where Mary Liz was perched in the baby seat.

"Hi, gorgeous", he said, reaching for her hand.

"Don't talk to strangers, Mary", I said.

"My name's Greg, and I think you're lovely", he said. The baby beamed at him. "She really is beautiful", he said.

You're not bad yourself, I thought. But being a respectable, middle-aged matron, I just smiled and thanked him.

And that's what happens all the time. Young and old, their faces light up when they see the baby coming. Her Majesty the Baby. Babyhood is the only time in a person's life that he is loved unconditionally even by strangers. A baby doesn't have to be witty or educated or interesting or good looking. He doesn't have to be virtuous or industrious or earn a living. He just sits and dribbles, and people think he's marvelous. But there must be more to it than that . . . I wonder if the baby, being a temple of the Holy Spirit, represents the sweetness and innocence of God and if that is what attracts people so powerfully.

And now I must finish this book before my slave master awakens and cracks the whip. She is a few feet away as I write, flaked out, legs akimbo in unladylike fashion, hair standing up in a mohawk, fat cheeks puffed out contentedly. She is our master, we are her slaves. No master ever had more willing slaves. She drools and throws up all over us, and we are awed at how lovely she is. She dirties her diaper, and we say how brilliant she is. She wakes at 4 A.M., and we're cooing because she smiles at us, a big, tonsil-baring smile that says, "Hi, guys! I recognize you!"

And so I finish where I began, my heart prostrate in thanksgiving for prayers heard and answered. You are our God. There is no other God like you. Because you have made me a mother and given me the joy of motherhood, I praise you with another mother's words. They are the words of a mother who was pregnant and thrilled to be so, a mother whom you yourself cherished with an infant's love: "My soul proclaims the greatness of the Lord. My spirit rejoices in God my savior, for he has looked with favor on his lowly servant. . . . The Almighty has done great things for me and holy is his name" (Lk 1:46–49).

For my baby's smile, for the blue of her eyes, for the tiny arms clinging to my neck—I praise you. Thank you, Father; thank you, Jesus; thank you, Holy Spirit.

Postscript

My story has ended. Or has it? When Mary Liz was twelve months old and this diary was in the process of going to press, a strange thing happened. I found I was pregnant again! Our fifth little angel is due the day after my forty-fourth birthday. When I was writing this diary, I was an old pregnant woman; now I'm an antique. God has a sense of humor, doesn't he? We are all thrilled, and once again we say, "Thank you, Lord, for the precious gift of life."

Notes

Notes

Notes

Notes

Notes

Notes